Living and Learning wi

A Guide for Parents and Teachers
of Visually Impaired Children

Blind and visually impaired children experience the world in unique ways. To help them learn and develop, parents and teachers need to understand how such children relate to their environment. Felicity Harrison and Mary Crow, who have spent years working with blind children and their families, offer practical strategies for encouraging the blind child's development and interaction with his or her family and school community.

The authors begin by discussing the reactions of parents when they learn their child is visually impaired, perhaps even multihandicapped. They go on to provide insights into what it means not to see well and techniques for encouraging the child to use whatever vision he or she may have. They suggest activities that parents or teachers can share with a blind child, from songs, games, and crafts to projects around the house and ways to enjoy a walk together. They discuss the nursery school experience and offer ideas on how to make it enjoyable and rewarding. A final chapter addresses preventive and remedial measures; it focuses on the nonvisual perspective and explains how to perceive things from the blind child's point of view.

Parents and preschool teachers of visually impaired children will find this a welcome guide to coping with day-to-day challenges and enhancing the child's education and development.

FELICITY HARRISON is Children's Consultant with the Canadian National Institute for the Blind, and volunteer Co-founder and Program Director of the Daylight Centre.

MARY CROW is Co-ordinator of the Infant Development Program, Ontario Foundation for Visually Impaired Children.

Living and Learning with Blind Children

A Guide for Parents and Teachers of Visually Impaired Children

FELICITY HARRISON
and
MARY CROW

UNIVERSITY OF TORONTO PRESS
Toronto   Buffalo   London

© University of Toronto Press Incorporated 1993
Toronto   Buffalo   London
Printed in Canada

ISBN 0-8020-2826-8 (cloth)
ISBN 0-8020-7700-5 (paper)

Printed on acid-free paper

Canadian Cataloguing in Publication Data

Harrison, Felicity.
  Living and learning with blind children

  Includes bibliographical references and index.
  ISBN 0-8020-2826-8 (bound). ISBN 0-8020-7700-5 (pbk.)

  1. Children, Blind. 2. Visually handicapped
  children. I. Crow, Mary, 1933– . II. Title.

  HV1596.2.H37 1993   362.4′18   C92-095308-5

Photos by Sharon Barnes (page 117), Mary Crow (pages 44, 95, 118, 123,
124, 129, 130, 134, 164, 166), Felicity Harrison (pages 84, 187), and Kevin
Stewart (pages 23, 33, 99, 190, 191, 192). Diagrams by Felicity Harrison.

Cover photograph by Ruth Naylor

Contents

Acknowledgments   vii

Introduction   3

1 Expectations and Attitudes   6

2 The Early Years and Steps to Independence   30

3 The Forty Points   83

4 Functional Vision and Creating Visual Interest   107

5 Practical Learning Experiences   120

6 Action Songs and Chants   144

7 Games and Crafts   152

8 Walks and Story-telling   188

9 Nursery School and Kindergarten   205

10 Preventive and Remedial Measures   216

Bibliography   263

Index   265

Acknowledgments

We would like to thank the Hospital for Sick Children Foundation, Toronto, for generous financial support in the preparation of this guide. The Foundation subsequently made a further generous grant towards the initial costs of publication, specifically to make the book more readily available to individuals who may benefit from it.

We would also like to thank The Canadian National Institute for the Blind, Ontario Division, for their cooperation and support in allowing Felicity a few months' leave of absence to start the project and for the ongoing use of equipment and facilities.

Special thanks to the blind and visually impaired children and their families who have been the inspiration for our work. Over the past twenty years their experiences, thoughts, and comments, both immediate and in retrospect, have been woven into the anecdotes and ideas expressed in this book.

Thank you to the readers who critiqued our manuscript and to the co-workers, friends, and relatives who with their questions and encouragement have made us think and rethink our material.

Over the years so many people have helped and spurred us on that it is impossible to name them all. However, it would be remiss of us not to give special mention to the following people: Jane Eacott and Richard Westgate, who spent many hours deciphering our handwriting, typing our material, and, later, transferring it onto computer; Geoffrey Harrison, who did the initial editing; and Mike and Eileen Harrison, Stephen Harrison (music), Reta McWhinnie, and Grace Fick, who all helped us meet deadlines.

Living and Learning
with Blind Children

Introduction

The vast majority of adults seldom think of visual impairment. When they do it is likely to be in relation to the elderly, who may have failing eyesight, or to children in Third World countries, who are blind as the result of malnutrition or disease. A passing encounter with a visually impaired person may raise brief speculation on what life without sight might be like. A blind person who is striding confidently down the street, white cane moving purposefully to ensure a safe route, can elicit our admiration for overcoming his or her disability, while the sight of a helpless blind beggar may elicit our pity. In either situation these brief speculations may be coloured by past experience and perhaps deep-rooted cultural concepts of blindness. Thus the subconscious mental image formed about blindness may have little bearing on reality and none at all on the needs of a visually impaired child. Through these pages we hope you will meet and learn about blind and partially sighted children. Geoffrey is one.

> Geoffrey stood alone, humming. Some distance from him the rest of the grade one class talked excitedly, pretending to be the TV crew who had visited their classroom the previous day. Fearing her blind student was feeling left out, the teacher said, 'Geoffrey, the others are having fun pretending. Why don't you join them?' 'I am,' Geoffrey said in surprise. 'I'm the camera!'

As you can see, visually impaired children will not have the same perception of the world as their sighted contemporaries. It may not be better or worse, but it will be different. They have the same basic needs as sighted children. Their potential to learn is comparable, but their method of learning is different. Sighted children see the whole at a glance and then may look at detail. In contrast, visually impaired children must first explore the details before they can understand the whole. The sighted child sees at a glance what is in the room, then chooses where to focus attention. Visually impaired children may be aware of only their immediate environment, the object with which they are in contact, or the noises around them. Sound, touch, smell, and taste are all important factors of the integration process. Without sight, the other sensory experiences, especially sound, are often disconnected. Even though an impression is formed, it will not be understood until a connection has been made. At the preschool level verbal information alone is not sufficient unless a concrete experience has preceded it.

In this book we have chosen to use the pronoun 'he.' This simplifies both the writing and reading and is less confusing than changing from one gender to another or using both simultaneously as 'he/she.' All anecdotal situations are true. However, names are fictitious and, in a few cases, circumstances or details have been altered to prevent identification or confusion.

A person is considered blind if the visual acuity in the better eye (with proper refractive lenses) is 20/200 or less. This means that even with glasses or contact lenses the person can see only at 20 feet (6 m) or less what could normally be seen at 200 feet (60 m). A person is also considered blind if the greatest diameter of the field of vision in both eyes is less than twenty degrees, in which case the person has tunnel vision.

Throughout this book, the term 'visual impairment' will be used to refer to any child who is blind as defined above. At times, it will be necessary to differentiate between totally blind and partially sighted. The word 'blind' refers to a child with minimal or no vision, and 'partially sighted' to a child with useful residual vision, but who still falls into the defined category of blindness.

Our goal is to help you understand how the visually impaired child learns all about the world. It is just as difficult for the sighted adult to relate to the world of the visually impaired child as it is for the preschool visually impaired child to learn about the sighted world. Together the child and the adult need to grow in their understanding.

We have offered guide-lines, made practical suggestions, and highlighted potential problem areas. Our intention is to give our readers a wide information base from which to draw. We hope this base will increase their understanding and give them confidence to think through ways of interacting with visually impaired children and plan their own course of action. Visually impaired children are as unique and individual as sighted children. What works for one may not be at all effective for another.

If the amount of information in this book seems overwhelming, remember it covers a diverse group of children and not all information will be pertinent to any one child. Above all, we would like this book to help the parents and families of visually impaired pre-schoolers share experiences and enjoy each other.

ONE

Expectations and Attitudes

All children need love, food, and shelter. An equally important need is a positive self-image. Learning to be independent is a step in achieving this.

Independence in small children is frequently thought of in terms of skills the child has learned in areas of self-help, language, and socialization. For example, can the child undress, dress, or feed himself? Is he toilet-trained? Does he express his needs and can he be understood by those other than his family? Does he shy away from or interact with other children? These are important, but there are other aspects of independence. Confidence is only one.

The dictionary has many definitions of independence, including autonomy and self-reliance. If a visually impaired child is to learn about himself and his environment, he will require more guidance than a child who can see, and this in turn can easily foster dependence on the person who is guiding him. For our purpose, the word 'independence' has greater meaning when read as 'dependence on self.' The meaning is the same – only the emphasis is different. The very nature of visual impairment affects a visually impaired child's opportunities for self-dependence. There are subtle areas of independence or dependence on self that parents and teachers of sighted children seldom have to consider. For example, when is a person on his own? What constitutes separation from others?

It is important to note that in certain situations a blind child may only *appear* to be independent. The child may be observed playing happily in part of a room or even in another room, seemingly absorbed in what he is doing and oblivious to what is going on around him. In reality the child may be as tuned in to his parent or teacher as a sighted child who is playing, but who is also watching and aware of the movements of an adult. The blind child may not perceive himself as being alone or separate from others.

> Totally blind four-and-a-half-year-old Christine was in nursery school. She was at the far end of a very large room playing with other children in the housekeeping corner, which was divided by a bookcase from the central open area of the classroom. It was a free-play period, so there was a general buzz of noise. At the other end of the room, the classroom teacher spoke to a small boy. 'Better pick that up or someone will fall over it,' she told him. Christine, who was busy playing at the toy stove, stopped what she was doing and said, 'Oh, okay,' then felt around on the floor and picked up a cereal box.

The sighted children in the housekeeping corner had tuned out the noises from the other side of the bookcase, which was a visual barrier. Behind it, they were in their own little room. What happened on the other side was of little concern to them because they were relating to the area they could see. The bookcase was not a visual barrier for Christine, so she was still tuned in to her teacher at the other side of the room, while acting in the same way as her sighted companions in the housekeeping corner.

Separation or full independence will have different implications, depending on whether a child is blind or sighted. If a child is sighted, separation will depend primarily on whether or not the child *sees* anyone with him. For a blind child, separation will depend primarily on whether or not the child *hears* anyone with him. Here is a list of points that indicate ways in which a sighted child's independence can be increased. Dependency on self in the sighted preschool child is apparent and developing when:

- parents' expectations of themselves are realistic
- others' expectations of the child are realistic
- the child's expectations of himself are realistic
- attitudes do not impose unnecessary limitations
- the child can imitate others
- the child can relate to environmental information
- the child can solve problems and has opportunities to make and correct mistakes
- there are challenging opportunities

- the child can communicate meaningfully
- there are opportunities to compare himself with others

We will explore each of these points, and as we do so the special needs of a visually impaired child will become evident. No one point stands on its own, but each interacts and overlaps with the others.

Realistic Expectations

The expectations of a visually impaired child's family and teachers for themselves and for him all affect his ability to achieve self-dependence. The adults' expectations will be reflected in the expectations the child has for himself. This section will explore these interconnected expectations.

When an infant is born with a disability, parents are usually totally unprepared for and may even be scared by the depth of their own emotions and those of their loved ones, which may be conflicting, confusing, and totally out of character. The following are just a few of the common emotions parents experience.

Constant weeping. A mother said, 'I had been accused of being unemotional. I seldom cried. When Claire was born, I couldn't stop, I didn't know what was happening to me. When she was six months old, I found myself crying because I'd burned a casserole. Things like that had always been just part of the ups and downs of a normal day.'

Confusion. One parent recalled a bewildering combination of anger, sorrow, and love. 'After Janice was born, I'd sometimes look at her and feel really angry. I'd even feel angry with her, I couldn't believe it of myself. She was so pretty, so weak, and so dependent on me. I felt very confused. I'd fluctuate from anger to an overwhelming sorrow and love for her.'

Blame. Many people struggle to find out why their baby has a problem. They try to find out what they or the doctor did or did not do, or they wonder if someone else is blaming them, as one woman describes it. 'My husband was a strong person. Nothing seemed to upset him, yet when Gerry was born I thought he was cracking up. I wanted him to hold me, but somehow I felt he didn't even want to touch me. I thought he was blaming me for Gerry's blindness.'

Hurt and shame. Friends and loved ones don't always understand. Sometimes their efforts to help can be very hurtful, one mother reported. 'Peter was a year old when my best friend said, "You've got to snap out of this nonsense. Go to the doctor. Maybe you need a tonic. I'm tired of your gloom. Your son is beautiful and you should be ashamed to carry on like this. I can't believe it – it's so unlike you." I hated her that day. What did she know about my reactions? Her daughter wasn't blind. But mostly I hated her because she echoed what I was already feeling about myself. She didn't know it, but I had been to the doctor. I was tired and ashamed of myself. Nothing seemed to be helping. I was scared. My feelings were out of control. At times I thought I was losing my mind.'

Inability to give emotional support. Fathers also experience emotions beyond their understanding, but sometimes their feelings are given less recognition. This can block communication between parents and cause great tension. A father said, 'I'd look at my wife. She seemed so crushed. I wanted to help her, but I couldn't. I resented my mother-in-law because my wife turned to her. I was supposed to be my wife's support, but I felt like a little boy who wanted to run away and hide. I wished I had parents to run to. I felt very much alone.'

Believing it to be a punishment from God. One father recalled thinking that the birth of his blind daughter was an act of divine retribution. 'My buddy and I were both expecting our babies on the same day. We kidded each other about whose boy would be born first. I knew it would be mine. I would even have made a small bet on it. Then my daughter Farah was born, premature and blind. I felt so guilty that I thought it was a punishment from God for wanting my child born first, and for wishing so much for a boy. I couldn't tell my wife because I knew I was being ridiculous, but the thought wouldn't go away. I didn't even tell them at the office when Farah was born. My buddy's son arrived on the expected day. I should have picked up the phone and congratulated him, but just couldn't do it. I didn't know why and I felt really badly, especially as he'd phoned me when Farah was born.'

Unreasonableness, irritability, and a need for recognition. Another father reported venting his emotions on his young son. 'I found myself being very irritable and unreasonable with my family after David was born. It was mostly about things that were totally unimportant. I wanted to comfort my wife and be the strong father I believed myself to be. It bothered me that I couldn't do it. One Saturday my four-year-old son asked when we were going to the river. I always took him on Saturdays. He looked forward to it. I told him we wouldn't go because I didn't feel like it. It was as if I wanted him to understand and be sorry for me. Eventually I took him because he looked so hurt, but he didn't have any fun. I was irritable and knew he was not to blame, but that seemed to make it worse, not better. I grumbled at him for silly things that normally we'd have laughed about. Those were dreadful days sometimes. Now they seem so far away, and yet at other times, they seem like yesterday.'

Disguised or delayed feelings and the search for miraculous cures. Many parents go to great lengths to find a new cure or someone to help them and their child. Sometimes, even after logic and reason tell them the search is futile, they feel compelled to continue. Great demands are often made on the family in the early days and months, such as medical emergencies or, equally stressful, a suspected but unconfirmed problem. At times parents are under so much stress that they appear to be living on adrenaline alone. When this happens, the disturbing but very normal reactions tend to submerge, only to surface much later. One grandmother said, 'My son and daughter-in-law were wonderful when Paul was born. He was multihandicapped and had very little vision. They seemed to live in and out of hospitals. Jenny was always so positive and brave, and my son too. When my grandson was two-and-a-half years old, his parents cancelled a long-anticipated trip abroad in order to vacation instead in a town where a faith healer was holding meetings. Previously, they thought faith healers were nothing more than charlatans. Only then did I know how badly they were still feeling inside. I felt sad that I had not recognized how much hurt they were hiding.'

Each person is unique and will react in his or her own way to the birth of a disabled infant. To try to understand the trauma and emotions, such as those described above, it is necessary to look back to before the baby was born. Those powerful and sometimes puzzling emotions originate before the baby's birth, and that too is where parents' expectations begin.

Preparing for an infant is usually a joyous and exciting period. It is also an emotional and very tiring time, especially if parents are expecting their first baby. The normal chores still need to be attended to, but now there is extra work to be done, and for the mother-to-be, the added weight of a growing infant doesn't make it any easier. There are choices and decisions to be made, shopping and perhaps rearranging the home to accommodate the new little one. There may also be an added strain on the budget. The prevailing emotion, however, is usually one of eager anticipation. This happy feeling can override the stress from the preparation, planning, and extra work. Many a pregnant woman wonders why she is so tired. 'I eat right, rest, in fact I do just what the doctor ordered,' she says, 'but at the end of the day I'm worn out.' Young women, who were previously able to dance all night, find themselves falling into bed at nine! Excitement and anticipation can also cause fatigue. Of course, there are always some who sail through pregnancy, full of vigour and energy. Although it may not be obvious, they too will experience stress as they prepare for the new arrival, and contemplate the changes it will mean in their immediate future.

Pregnancy is a time when thoughts turn to parental skills, and new parents-to-be may wonder about what kind of parents they want to be and how they plan to achieve their goals. One mother said, 'After my grandma died, I remembered how much I missed our "quiet times," as she called them. She would make up or read stories to me and we'd just chat. That period was very special. When I was expecting my first child, I decided that I would make the time before bedtime very special for our child. I planned that this time together would be a priority.'

A father told how he had not had the opportunity to appreciate and know his own father until he was at university. He was determined that his child would have a real dad, someone to know, love, and respect. From the beginning, he decided he would take time to be with his child. Another mother spoke of how serious she was when her baby was due. For her, having a baby was a special privilege. She'd waited for a baby for many years. She said, 'I imagined a book with blank white pages. This was my baby's life. I felt a great responsibility. I would be one of the scribes who would write on those pages. I wanted each page to be very special, to read like a beautiful poem.'

Work, plans, choices, decisions, expectations, goals, and dreams are all woven into the fabric of the time before an infant arrives. The long-awaited day comes, the tension mounts, and finally the baby is born. Then immediately, or over a period of time, parents learn that something is wrong. The baby is not the baby they expected. Expectations, goals, and dreams all seem shattered. Nothing makes sense any more. They feel battered and bruised and life becomes a struggle. A sibling's school essay may be an oversimplification, perhaps, but it sums up the situation very well.

'It's like looking through a catalogue, deciding on what to order, placing the order, and waiting excitedly for it to arrive. Then when it comes, opening the parcel and finding it isn't what you ordered. You feel a great disappointment. You cry and become angry. You want to send it back and get the right order, but you can't because the company went out of business. That makes you want to stamp and shout, you feel so frustrated, but it doesn't do any good. Then after a while you look again at the parcel. It's not what you ordered, but it is very nice, and you find you actually like it. Then something happens: it becomes very special. My sister is like such a parcel. She's different, but I love her very much.'

Grief and turmoil are a shock to the body, and the whole family system has taken an emotional beating. Just as the reactions of each person differ, the healing process for each person will also be different. There is some truth in the old adage 'Time heals.' The following wise advice from other parents may be helpful.

'Be patient with yourself and your loved ones. They want to help but may not know how. Take it a day at a time. You don't believe it, but life does become normal again. Accept it from one who knows.'

'Don't expect to be able to communicate immediately, but try to keep the doors of communication open. I wanted to talk about it, but my husband seemed almost indifferent. I didn't understand that he too was grieving. It nearly cost us our marriage. When he was able to talk I shut him out. We understand each other now and are stronger for it.'

'Some days I thought I'd go crazy. There were so many friends and professionals telling me what to do. There always seemed to be appointments. Someone was coming to the house or I was going to them. Doctors, therapists, counsellors, and friends. I seemed to be on a treadmill and I didn't know how to get off. My five-year-old son stopped the treadmill. All he said was, "Don't you love us any more, Mom?" His little face looked up at me at that moment and shocked me back to reality. I realized that the baby, even though she had special needs, was not a priority. Our whole family was priority, and she was part of it. I hadn't realized I was allowing her to separate us. When I re-evaluated my activities, I found that some appointments were unnecessary, while others could be rearranged. Everything changed when I forced myself to say no to outside demands and took time just to be alone with my family. I worried that my baby would regress. What surprised me most was that the baby, instead of regressing, became more relaxed and much stronger. We all began to enjoy her and each other. My advice is to give yourself time to relax with your husband and children, and the baby will benefit from it. Your baby needs a real family to be part of.'

'Don't be scared to use the words "blind" or "visually impaired" when talking about your child. They are not dirty words. Sometimes I found this very difficult, but when I started to say the words, they didn't seem so terrible, and I found that other people relaxed and seemed more comfortable with us.'

'The best advice I had was from my husband. It was some months after our son was born. I had had a particularly discouraging week. I had worked hard with my son and was very tired. He wasn't progressing the way I felt he should. I found myself in tears or irritable and snapping at my family. On this particular day, my husband came in after work on Friday. "I've made plans for tomorrow," he announced. "I know you planned to do the laundry and clean the house while I did the shopping. I was able to get off work early and I've done the shopping. What I've missed doing we can do together tomorrow. Esther is coming to look after the baby at 9:30 in the morning. She's a nurse, she loves babies, and will know what to do if he has a seizure. I'm taking you out," and he added, "Esther said she'd do the laundry."

'My poor husband. I remembered bursting into tears, I shouted at him that he had no right to make plans for me without consulting me. I'll never forget his words or his loving expression. "You know," he said as he firmly held my shoulders, "you are very important to me. Remember, you are my wife, my lover, my best friend, and you are the mother of our child. You are very valuable to me. I want you to value yourself highly. I don't want you to become broken or worn down. You need time for yourself, and I'd hoped you'd want to share some of it with me."

'My husband knew me better than I knew myself. I did need time away. Together we had a wonderful day. Over the years I've needed the help of friends and professionals, and now I'm in a position to help others. I believe the advice of my husband is still the best advice I could have had and I'm glad to pass it on. Value yourself highly. You are important.'

Who better to give direction than those who've travelled the road before? You are important. Value yourself highly. Be patient. Take time to heal. This is wise advice. Many parents have such high expectations of themselves that healing becomes very difficult. Unfortunately, friends and professionals often unwittingly augment this problem by giving advice on how to help the baby progress. When parents already feel a great burden to do everything they can for their infant, they struggle to follow any advice, even asking for more. Then they feel guilty if they don't reach the standard that they believe is expected of them or that they have set for themselves. Instead of learning to love and communicate with their new little one, the prevailing theme becomes 'Work with the baby.' Cherishing and love take second place. In those first few months, with very few exceptions, the baby's greatest need is for cherishing, not 'being worked with.' To be cuddled and, yes, even washed by a parent's tears. The security of loving arms helps the infant relax and grow stronger, and in turn allows the parents the necessary time to recover.

Stress can be like an insidious mist. It creeps up and then enfolds, to become a dense fog. There seems no way out, like the treadmill described earlier. Remembering to value yourself highly is excellent advice. No parent is a superman or superwoman. Body parts and nerves cannot be replaced like screwing a new bolt into a bionic arm, leg, or nerve. The whole body is tired. It must have rest. Negative stress can cause sickness, a broken marriage, or child abuse. Stress can change people, even those who are patient and normally stable. Parents need to recognize the signs and take action. Extended family or friends, if they are asked, may be willing to help. Pride must not get in the way of asking. Sometimes it is necessary to involve a professional.

As a visually impaired infant grows older, the need for assistance in helping him interpret and understand his world will increase, and so too will the demands on his family. Parents need to be aware that this will happen and begin early to prepare a relief system. Ideally, removing a little one to a program is not the answer. A visually impaired child's interests are best met in his own home or, if that is not possible, in a home setting. One creative family who had no extended family or friends nearby to help, advertised for a person or couple willing to act as grandparents for a visually impaired preschooler with additional handicaps. They received several replies. Not only did they find foster grandparents, they also made several new friends.

A father with five small daughters believed his wife should have a full day off each week. He treated it as a priority. He was not affluent, but by cutting back in other areas, he managed to pay some-one to care for the children biweekly. On the alternate weeks, a co-worker's wife with three older children took his five younger ones for a day. On the following day his wife looked after the three older children, giving their mother a free day. The older children enjoyed helping care for the little ones, and both families were happy with the arrangement.

Grieving is to be expected, and is part of the healing process. The conflicting emotions you are experiencing are normal. Time does heal, but be prepared for unexpected emotions to surface, even after you are feeling more like yourself again. They will occur less and less frequently, but they will happen. It will help if you are able to think your feelings through and understand them. It is also important that you allow yourself to seek help and accept it when it is offered, or refuse it if the help itself becomes stressful. Finally, try to determine whether the expectations you have for yourself and your family are realistic because if they are not, life for you and your family will be off balance, and this will affect the ongoing development of your visually impaired child.

Expectations Others Have for the Child

A realistic expectation can be described as the normal or average in any given situation. However, recognizing what is normal or average is often difficult. Attitudes, situations, experiences, visual ability, personality, and intelligence are many of the variables that colour the issue. Visual impairment creates its own special needs, but the total child and his environment must be considered. The following hypo-thetical situations may help to make this clearer.

Imagine the setting is a quiet street that ends at the school yard of a rural community school. There are no intersections and there are houses on either side of the street. Each house has one or more children who attend the community school. An average seven-year-old child could walk with schoolmates to the school. In the following situations, the first three children are sighted.

Situation 1: Attitudes. Sarah had always walked to school accompanied by her older brother and classmates. Just before term began, Sarah's older brother, in hot pursuit of a football, ran out onto the street. He didn't see or hear the mail truck slowly approaching the drive, and ran into it, ending up in hospital with a broken rib. Since the accident, Sarah's mother's attitude has changed. She now drives her daughter to school.

Situation 2: Judgment. Seven-year-old Lucy walks to school. One day, while playing in the yard, she trips over her bicycle and breaks her leg. She comes home from the hospital with a walking cast to the knee. Lucy is proud of her cast, asking everyone to sign it. To her family's surprise, Lucy continues her activities, seemingly oblivious of the added weight on one leg. Is it a realistic expectation that Lucy walk to school? One might argue that she should if she has no difficulty in continuing with her activities. Another person might counter-argue that the walk to school may be too long and therefore too demanding for Lucy. She might arrive at school on time, but may be too tired to work effectively. We now have a judgment situation. Lucy's mother must decide whether her daughter is strong enough to walk to school.

Situation 3: Emotional fragility. Seven-year-old Frieda was adopted when she was four years old. She has had serious health problems, but is now healthy. Physically she is small, emotionally fragile, and very immature. She lacks confidence, is timid and easily upset. She has not yet made friends. Frieda's mother walks her to school, and makes a special effort to chat with the other children so that they will want to join Frieda and herself. Frieda's mother and teacher are both working towards building Frieda's confidence and helping her to interact with her classmates. They believe that Frieda can walk to school without an adult. They are working towards that goal.

Situation 4: Confident personality. Terry is seven years old and totally blind. His family has recently moved into the neighbourhood. Terry attended grade one in another school. As they had lived in a big city, Terry was driven to school. He has already made friends with the neighbourhood children and finds his way independently to the neighbours' homes on both sides of the street. He frequently has to contend with a car parked in the driveway or bicycles left lying around. He has learned to use the phone and remembers the numbers of his friends. He can phone them completely independently. Terry is an unusually confident and self-assured little boy. Should Terry walk to school with his new friends? This is the dilemma for Terry's parents.

In making their decision they considered all aspects and decided that, apart from his lack of vision, Terry compared favourably in all other aspects with the neighbourhood children, and appeared even more mature than some. This itself, they decided, could be a problem. Terry is a determined, strong-willed little boy. He might not listen to his sighted friends. They want their son to lead a normal and independent life, but are also realistic and recognize his limitations. They decide that Terry should walk to school with his schoolmates. They realize that to prepare him will demand time and energy. They decide Terry must first learn the route. Over the next few days Terry, his mother, and sometimes his father walk from their home to the school and back. They talk about the terrain, different sounds, and landmarks. His mother encourages Terry to tell her what he is noticing. Keeping on the sidewalk, Terry follows the borders of the neighbours' gardens. Soon Terry was ready to try walking the route independently. On his trial walk, Terry makes two mistakes. He turns too soon and goes up the driveway of a house, thinking it is the school yard, but he corrects himself. Next, he has difficulty finding the school gate and becomes angry. Terry and his mother discuss how they can overcome this problem. 'I know,' she says, 'you can go from the mailbox to the big tree.' 'What big tree?' Terry asks. His mother shows him. It was just behind the mailbox. 'If you stand with your back against the mailbox and feel the big tree on your left, you will be in just the correct position. Now if you walk forward, you will come to the school gate and won't have to go all around the curve.' Terry was enthusiastic. The first time he tried on his own, he found the big tree, but did not position himself correctly and missed the gate. The next time, he placed his back to the mailbox, found the gate with ease, and was very pleased with himself. Soon Terry walks the route with no difficulty.

Terry's parents discuss his progress. 'I am just not sure how Terry will do if he gets excited and interested in other children's conversation, or if the children run off and leave him. I wonder if he isn't subconsciously depending on me. He surprises me, he is so tuned in to my every move.' After further discussion, Terry's father decided he will take Terry and tell him while they are walking about an upcoming vacation to Grandma's.

Terry and his father set out. Terry is thrilled when his father tells him of the upcoming trip and chats excitedly, never once losing track of the route. Terry's father says, 'Just listen to the birds and the noises around. We'll walk in silence.' Without telling Terry, he steps onto the grass and starts to take very big steps. Soon he is well ahead of his son. Almost immediately Terry is aware that his father is not beside him and calls out. 'Daddy!' he shouts anxiously. 'Dad! Dad!' No reply. Terry moves back and forth, shouting for his father. Hardly able to keep from speaking, Terry's father watches in silence and continues to watch as his son's lip trembles and he starts to cry. Once more Terry shouts for his father and listens. Then Terry turns and runs towards home. 'Mom!' he shouts, 'Where's Dad?'

Terry's father picks him up. 'You've passed my test, Terry,' he said as he hugs him. 'You stayed on the route, even though you were excited, and you found your way home when you thought you were lost. Now I know you'll be okay. On Monday you can walk to school with your pals. I am so proud of you.' Terry stops crying and a big smile stretches across his face.

The prerequisites have been met. It is now a realistic expectation for Terry to walk to school with his friends. The experiences and practice provided Terry with invaluable learning opportunities.

Situation 5: Change in routine. Bonny and Beth are seven-year-old identical twins. Beth is partially sighted, but her serious visual impairment is not obvious, especially as both children wear glasses. The twins have older brothers, Steven and Michael, aged ten and twelve. Although inseparable, the girls are very sociable and neighbourhood children frequently visit. Bonny tends to be the leader in large groups and all active games. Beth is quieter and may seem shy. In an open space, it is usually Bonny who leads and Beth who follows. Inside the house, however, Beth is the leader, initiating the activity, which is frequently playing at housekeeping or school. The twins both enjoy construction toys. Bonny creates houses, towers, and bridges, in keeping with her panoramic view of the world, while Beth, relating to what she can most easily see, builds tables, chairs, and beds for her Barbie dolls.

The twins walk to school, usually with one or more friends. One day Bonny is sick and has to stay at home. Beth starts off confidently with the other children. Four houses along they come out from under the shade of the trees and Beth stops and seems confused. The other children are skipping along and chatting and don't realize that Beth is not with them. When they turn, they are surprised to see that she is crying behind them.

Beth had stopped to find her sunglasses, which she carries in her lunch-box, but the catch was stuck. She called for Bonny, but then remembered Bonny was still at home. Her friends, although not far away, were too far for Beth to see. Beth had become frightened and started to cry. In bright light, without her sunglasses, Beth could see very little. Previously when Bonny was close by, this was not a problem. Beth just kept close beside her until they were in the less sunny area.

The next day, although Bonny was still sick, her mother decided Beth should walk to school. She used this situation as an opportunity to help Beth explain her visual impairment to her friends. 'It's like when you are driving in the car and the windshield is dirty, but it doesn't look dirty until the sun shines and then the driver can hardly see to drive and has to use the windshield washers.' Beth's mother had explained. Steven's friend said, 'I didn't know you couldn't see very well, Beth. I'll walk with you to school until Bonny is better.'

Situation 6: Multihandicapped. Rochelle, who is seven years old and has cerebral palsy, is severely visually impaired. She can take a few steps independently, but needs a wheelchair for any distance travel. Her understanding of language is good, but her speech is often difficult to understand.

Rochelle attends a special class in the local school. At home Rochelle is encouraged to do as much as possible for herself, e.g., moving herself from the family room to the dining-room at mealtime by walking, crawling, or shuffling.

Rochelle's mother has always pushed her to school in her wheel-chair. Now twelve-year-old Jean, one of the neighbourhood girls who frequently walks with them, has asked if she can take Rochelle to school every morning. Rochelle seems to be excited by the idea. The parents weigh the pros and cons: Jean and Rochelle enjoy each other's company; Jean is a reliable and sensible girl. Will Jean get tired of pushing Rochelle to school every day? Will Rochelle be hurt if this happens? Will Rochelle feel comfortable going to school without her mother, who realizes it will probably be more difficult for her than for Rochelle? They decide to give it a trial period and suggest that Jean may like to take Rochelle to school three days a week instead of five.

To sum up, for the visually impaired child, independence or dependency on self is achieved through realistic expectations. Use as a base the closest norm of the non-handicapped child. Then it is necessary to think it through and consider all the implications.

Expectations of the Child for Himself

The host of the TV program 'Tiny Talent Time' often asks his young guests, 'What would you like to be when you grow up?' Even the very smallest children have answers. Sometimes their answers are amusing, but usually they have been well thought out within the limits of the child's experiences and interest.

To think realistically about his future goals, the visually impaired child needs to have a positive self-image. This can only happen if those around him have a healthy attitude regarding his visual impairment. 'Lorna says she's going to be a nurse when she grows up. Can I be a nurse?' A simple discussion about nursing will not only help the child understand a nurse's work, but may help him come to his own decisions based on sound facts. 'I wouldn't be able to be a nurse,' the child might say. 'I wouldn't know where to put the needle to give an injection.' That remark may indicate the child is coming to his own conclusions about nursing. The response might be, 'That's right, nursing might not be for you, but there are other things that nurses do that you can learn to do. You can learn to put on a bandage and learn about things that help make people better.'

Role-playing; helping to nurse a sick baby, grandparent, or pet; hearing stories about people doing things for others that make them feel better; and later simple quizzes such as 'How would you know someone had a cold?' 'What could you do if you had a sore throat?' 'What do hiccups sound like? What can you do about them?' – all serve to increase the child's knowledge and help him understand that there are many things he can learn and do.

Depending on the child's level of maturity and interest, he can be told about other careers in the medical field that are possible even for a totally blind person, such as physiotherapy. The child could also learn that nursing is not the only occupation that helps people. Social work is another example. In almost all fields there are jobs that the visually impaired child can do instead of the usual work sighted children think about.

Sometimes, in spite of your discussions about a more appropriate occupation, the visually impaired child still fantasizes about being a nurse, a pilot, or a taxi driver. This is normal. Sighted children also dream of being an astronaut, a ballet dancer, a trapeze artist, or a lion tamer, but in time come to realize that in reality none of these occupations may be possible for them. Visually impaired children will also recognize that there are some activities they cannot do.

Regardless of how capable, well adjusted, and competent the visually impaired child is, there are always some things he will never be able to do, however much he would want to. Driving a car is an obvious one.

Willis, totally blind, tells of how his father's foresight helped him over this difficult period in his teens. When he was young his father made him aware of all the things young boys talk about. He learned about cars and how they differ from one another. He recalls happy outings with his dad spent in car lots, followed by his choice of restaurants. Every year he learned more. He learned to fill the gas tank and check the oil when he was still in kindergarten. Over the years he learned about engines. His father didn't know how to repair cars, so he asked his brother to teach him. From his uncle Willis learned to repair many things and often his sighted friends would ask his advice.

In his late teens he began dating girls and on his birthday his father bought him a second-hand car. 'Keep it in good repair and you can ask your girlfriend or buddy to drive it,' he was told. Willis was thrilled. His girlfriend later became his wife.

For those with difficulty thinking about what their child could possibly do, the *Survey of Occupations: Examples of Jobs Being Performed by Blind and Visually Impaired Canadians*, published by the national office of the Canadian National Institute for the Blind (CNIB), offers the following:

Canadians with little or no sight are successfully employed in a multitude of occupations and are represented in most of the major occupational groups, such as managerial, social sciences, teaching, medicine, clerical, sales – and many others. In this book you will find the job description of an industrial relations manager, comedian, clinical psychologist, laundry worker, nuclear engineering technologist, fisherwoman, florist and hog farmer, to name a few. The diversity of these career choices suggests that traditionally held views about the kinds of occupations which can be done by people with vision handicaps are inappropriate today.

It is important that the child's questions are always answered simply and honestly. To tell him that when he is older, he can do anything his sighted friends can does not help him to face reality. He will quickly learn that this is not true and may feel disappointed. He may then wonder about other things that he has been told, or question his own ability, feelings that perhaps he is not even as capable as other visually impaired children. The parents of one blind child, hoping to protect her, had always been overly reassuring in what they told her and in the answers they gave to her questions. When she was twelve years old she told her parents, 'I'm not really sure about what you say. You tell me these things because you love me.' An encouraging but always honest approach is preferable. Children are very perceptive and quickly recognize cover-ups or diverting tactics.

It is through day-to-day activities that realistic expectations are developed in a child. Do not always deprive the child of an opportunity to fail. It is only through experiencing failures and successes that he is able to realistically assess his abilities. It is an ongoing process. How you help your child deal with failures can build or shatter his confidence to try again.

Petra was attending her first day camp. She was a bright little girl with very limited vision. She had recently begun orientation and mobility training and was very proud of her new cane. On the third day when she arrived at camp with her mother, Mrs Downey, she boasted, 'I can find my own group,' and ran off without waiting for her mother. Seconds later Mrs Downey say Petra heading for a picnic table. She called, 'Petra, stop!' Petra did not listen and crashed into the table.

Mrs Downey might have physically stopped Petra from running off, or scolded her for running off and not listening, or felt guilty about what happened and rushed immediately to Petra's aid. Any of these actions would have been justifiable, but Mrs Downey recognized this as a valuable learning experience for her daughter and resisted reacting immediately. She walked over to her daughter and in a calm, concerned

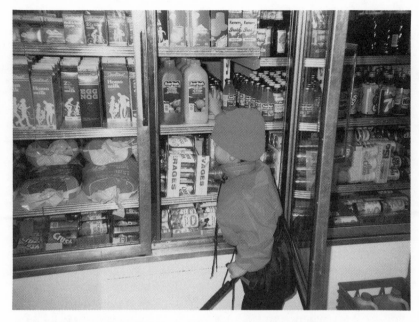

A reward for good work on an orientation and mobility lesson.

voice said, 'Are you okay, Petra?' Mrs Downey checked for scratches and bruises and reassured her.

Mrs Downey did not get cross with Petra or criticize what she had done. Instead she encouraged Petra to talk about what happened and why. Then she reminded Petra how well she had been doing in her mobility lessons, and that it is important for her to listen and concentrate. With directions from Mrs Downey, Petra then walked carefully and had no problems locating her group. Mrs Downey had allowed Petra to fail. Petra still experienced her mother's concern, but had an opportunity to learn through cause and effect. Through non-critical discussion, a reminder of her strengths, and an immediate opportunity to try again, Petra was encouraged and her self-esteem remained intact.

Talking about a child's blindness in a matter-of-fact way is important. He should be able to relate the words 'blind' and 'visually impaired' to himself. It helps him become comfortable with those words. Avoiding the use of the words or any discussion of his disability can cause the child to feel inferior and less confident in himself. When blind children ask about their eyes or about sight, they are often quite satisfied when they are told that they can't see with their eyes, but they can see with their hands. However, even this comment can sometimes require further explanation.

> Mary tells of Anna, a bright, totally blind six-year-old, who has to touch things with her hands in order to 'see' them and assumed everyone else did too. They talked about body parts and growing, about long arms and short arms, big hands and small hands, and how everyone was a little different. Mary explained that she could see with her eyes because she was sighted. However, being blind meant that the eyes did not work. Anna was blind and used her fingers to 'see.' Mary explained she could see with her eyes things that were close or far away without touching them, just as Anna could hear things close or far away without touching them. Mary recalled that Anna was quite satisfied with the explanation.

Even though the differences and limitations of blindness have been accepted at home, the issues may still come up at school. Other children will ask such questions as, 'Why are you blind?' 'How come you can't see when your eyes are open?' 'Why do your eyes look like that?' A visually impaired child needs answers. It is helpful if the child has the answers ready to use when needed, such as, 'I was born blind,' or 'This is the way they were when I was born,' or 'The insides of my eyes aren't working, so the outsides look different.' A question such as 'Will your eyes get better?' can be answered matter-of-factly, 'No, this is the way they are.' The answers should be short, honest, and straightforward. Children ask questions in a totally unabashed way, and they are equally quick to accept answers, particularly if the exchange is open and direct. One mother learned how needless her fears were and that children can accept disabilities quite readily.

> Vernon, who was born visually impaired, has facial marks and facial deformities. His mother said she dreaded sending her son to school. She would lie awake at night, wondering how the other children would treat him. 'Children can be so cruel,' she told herself, mistaking their natural curiosity and questions as cruelty. In spite of her fears, Vernon was treated very normally. The neighbours' children played with Vernon and his older sister. Vernon was a happy-go-lucky little boy. His ready, lopsided grin, cheerful personality, and laughter were infectious. When Vernon's mother left him in kindergarten that first day she

came home and wept bitterly, waiting fearfully for his return. Vernon came home all smiles. 'I've got a new friend,' he said. 'The kids asked me all kinds of questions about my face. We have a sharing time and the teacher let me tell them about all the times I go to hospital. They asked so many questions. I let my new friend try on my glasses. He said they felt funny, and he told me my face looked like I'd got paint on it. He makes me laugh. I can swing higher than he can. I like school.'

As Vernon's mother told herself, children can be cruel. The remark regarding paint on Vernon's face could have been hurtful. Several things had helped to lessen the impact of this remark. In spite of his mother's own anxieties, she did not overprotect him but allowed Vernon to have normal experiences and interact with neighbourhood children. His sensitive teacher understood what would be helpful to Vernon in this new situation. Vernon's personality and ability to answer questions no doubt helped him very much on his first day at school, making it a very successful day.

The independence or dependency on self of a blind or visually impaired child can be achieved when those around him are positive and encouraging but always truthful when they give him information or answer his questions. Parents need to be prepared for the fact that there will be difficult times. Those parents who start early will make it easier for themselves and will help their child understand himself and develop realistic expectations.

Attitudes

Visually impaired five-year-old Joan and her mother were Christmas shopping. As the purchases piled higher in the shopping cart, Joan's mother complained, 'Now I can't see where I'm going.' 'It's okay, Mum,' Joan responded brightly, 'I can never see where I'm going.'

Joan had a healthy attitude towards her blindness. A child's progress is often determined by his own attitude and the attitudes of those who interact with him. From a congenitally blind child's perspective, he is a total child. There are no feelings of loss. Sight as the sighted understand it is unknown to him. The progress of a preschooler who had sight but loses it will also depend to a great extent on his attitude and the attitudes of those who interact with him. This child will feel some loss. However, most of these children adjust very quickly. The visually impaired child will be aware that there is a difference between himself and those who can see. It is to be expected, and indeed hoped, that this recognition will take place early in life. For the visually impaired child, this is a normal development that often occurs during the latter part of the preschool years. If those who interact with the child have nurtured his feelings of self-worth, discussed his questions in an honest and matter-of-fact way, the child will benefit and grow emotionally and, most important, will develop a positive self-image. It is no more traumatic for a visually impaired preschool child to accept his disability than it is for a sighted child to understand that his peers possess talents that he does not have. Joan's attitude is not exceptional. Acceptance is normal. As all normally developing children begin to understand themselves, they quickly learn the art of manipulation.

> Joan found her handicap to be a convenient tool. On one occasion, her mother told her, 'You'd better put that chewing-gum in the garbage.' 'I can't,' Joan replied, holding the gum out to her mother, 'I'm blind.' 'So you are,' her mother responded with a laugh, 'but it doesn't affect your hands or your feet. You know where the garbage is. Take it there.' With a giggle, Joan took the gum to the garbage!

This is not very different from a sighted child who says, 'You carry my coat, it's too heavy,' or the child who asks, 'Will you get it? It's too high, I can't reach it,' but who pulls the chair out and climbs up with no difficulty when asked to bring down the Halloween trick-or-treat bag.

There are times when the visually impaired child becomes frustrated or irritated by the limitations imposed on him by his visual impairment. How people deal with their limitations and face obstacles in their lives depends to a large extent on the attitudes they learned as children. Children form these attitudes early in life by patterning themselves after those around them. Have you ever listened to small children playing with dolls? What they have experienced in the home is expressed in their play, sometimes to the surprise or chagrin of the listening adult.

Faulty attitudes are often the reason why a visually impaired child does not realize his potential. People who try to identify with a visually impaired child may in reality not be identifying with the child at all. What they may be doing is identifying with their imagined feeling of loss. Their attitudes towards the child are then governed by these feelings and manifest themselves as pity, guilt, fear, overprotectiveness or overindulgence – all inappropriate and very debilitating for the child.

A nursery school class was given blindfolds to try on. The teacher was preparing them for the arrival of a new classmate who was blind. She was amazed at the insight of one four-year-old who said, 'It's not really like this, is it, 'cause I know what things are like.'

The child was right. Putting blindfolds on is a useful exercise to make points and to discover methods likely to be most helpful in teaching a visually impaired child a new skill, but it does not duplicate visual impairment. Vision integrates all the fragments of sensory information we receive. This is interpreted by the brain as a visual image. As soon as people imagine themselves without vision, they place themselves in a totally new dimension. They feel inadequate and unable to cope. They have relied on sight in virtually everything they have done and it is not surprising that imagining what it is like to be without sight results in a feeling of great loss. The congenitally visually impaired child does not experience this loss as his brain has never interpreted the same visual images. It is impossible for a person who has never known sight to understand what it is like to see. It is equally impossible for a sighted person to comprehend blindness from birth. While it is not possible for a sighted person to identify with visual impairment, it is possible to identify with the problem the child is having, due to the visual impairment.

Three-and-a-half-year-old Bobby was in nursery school. Snack time was over. His teacher told the children to sit on the mat for story time. Bobby stood up and hesitated for a moment. Noticing this, the teacher's aide said, 'I'll take you, Bobby. Come along with me.' After the story, the teacher remarked, 'There is no need to bring Bobby to the mat.' 'I thought I'd help him,' the aide responded. 'It must be so difficult for him when he cannot see.' 'Watch,' the teacher said and called, 'Bobby, would you mind doing an errand for me?' 'Okay,' said Bobby. He stood up and again hesitated, listening to locate his teacher's whereabouts. 'I'm at the desk,' the teacher said, noticing his hesitation. Bobby headed directly towards her. 'Would you mind taking this note to Miss White's class for me, Bobby?' Bobby took the note and headed off willingly. 'Go to the door and watch,' the teacher suggested to the aide. 'I see what you mean,' the aide said, returning. 'He is so confident he doesn't need my help.'

'Sometimes he does need your help,' the teacher smiled. 'What he doesn't need is your pity.' She continued, 'When Bobby first came to this school, we all fell into the same trap as you have done. We felt sorry for Bobby and one of us was always there to help him. After a few weeks, I realized that Bobby was making no progress. He seemed bored and not very happy. We had a meeting and asked his parents to come. They said, "We don't identify with Bobby's blindness because we cannot understand it. We tell and show Bobby how to do things and then we leave him alone and let him experiment for himself. It may take him several trials before he succeeds. Sometimes we may offer Bobby help; sometimes he asks for help." They explained that Bobby's methods of solving problems were often quite different from theirs. Bobby's mother noted that Bobby had refined his non-visual senses in a way that they had not had to do. Their common sense and matter-of-fact approach to Bobby's needs were refreshing. We learned from them that it was never a good idea to hover over Bobby, that he would do much better if we stood back. We've been trying to follow that advice and you've just witnessed Bobby in action. The problem was our attitude. Bobby is proof of how we've changed!'

All children need time for fun and relaxation, to share laughter and humour so that they can understand and be comfortable with it. If they are always having demands made on them, they may not want to face life, but may become introverted and shut the world out. Conversely, if no demands are made on them, they may not learn responsibility and self-worth, but instead become self-centred and ineffective. If visually impaired children are to grow into well-adjusted adults who are able to set realistic goals for themselves, they must have the opportunity to know themselves in many situations and experience their strengths and weaknesses. They need opportunities to make mistakes and learn from them. By being shown courtesy and consideration, each child will learn that he is considered an important and integral part of his family, school, or community, but he should not be given the impression that he is the centre of it.

When well-meaning people allow a visually impaired child to be an exception to rules and expectations, the child may develop an exaggerated idea of his own importance, or perhaps feel left out and worthless. As with any child, a visually impaired child who believes or acts as if the world revolves around him is likely to be very unpopular. It's not an easy task for the caregivers to balance the needs of family members when one member requires additional time and energy. The needs of each family member are different and none is more important than the other. If one can adopt this attitude, the balancing act becomes a little easier. There will be less guilt attached to taking time for oneself or for other family members.

For the visually impaired child, independence or self-dependence is to a large extent determined by attitudes – how the child is perceived or perceives himself. A child's visual impairment is often less of a problem than the faulty attitudes adopted from those around him.

TWO

The Early Years and Steps to Independence

Mealtime

Physical contact provides so many benefits. Whenever possible hold your baby as he drinks his bottle instead of propping him up in his crib or play-pen. Encourage your baby to put two hands on the bottle and later to hold it. Small plastic bottles are easier to hold. If you present the bottle from a slightly different position each time, the infant will not become programmed to expect things to appear in exactly the same place.

Many visually impaired children resist new tastes and textures. To prevent this problem, introduce the infant to different tastes before he starts solid food. You can dip a teaspoon in your own food as you eat it (no food, just the taste is on the spoon). Even an infant will have definite taste preferences. Instead of always relying on prepared baby foods, try blending your own foods so that your infant becomes accustomed to the tastes. This makes it easier to accustom him to the same table foods with a different texture. Constipation is frequently a problem for visually impaired children. There are two main reasons why this is so. There may be a lack of fibre in a child's diet because he resists changing to new textures – remember there is no visual appeal. Also, visually impaired children often are not aware of the many opportunities to be physically active and consequently do not exercise sufficiently.

When your child can sit in a high chair or on your lap at the table to eat, encourage him to hold the bowl or dish and explore what is in it. If he is blind, this is the only way he will know that food is in the dish. Finger feeding usually precedes using a spoon. Encourage your child to pick up food from his tray or dish. This gives him practice in moving food from dish to mouth. It also gives him opportunities to feel the different textures of food. Place the food in different places on the tray to encourage your child to search.

Learning to use a spoon is a slow process. Once the child is able to hold the spoon, help him to move the spoon to his mouth with as little hand-over-hand assistance as possible. At first only expect him to lift one or two spoonfuls to his mouth, leaving you to feed him the rest of the food. Once he has control, is holding the spoon firmly, and is ready to start the scooping process, a deep, straight-sided dish will be helpful. The child dips the spoon into the dish, slides it across the bottom and brings it up the side of the dish. If the dish has deep, straight sides, the spoon will be close to his mouth and less direction will be needed. Say 'Dip, slide, and into your mouth' or a similar phrase. The rhythm and words help. Children often say the words, which helps them think about what they are doing. When the child is beginning to use a spoon, we suggest that you have a second spoon ready and make sure he gets a mouthful of food each time he makes an attempt.

Encourage your child to use a cup, even though he may still drink from the occasional bottle or cup with lid and spout. To learn the tipping process, the cup needs to be filled to the top so that the blind child receives the immediate satisfaction of liquid on his lips. Any small container is useful here – one parent stuck several lightweight plastic eggcups together and filled the top one. (One small eggcup is difficult for child and parent to manipulate together.) This prevents wasting lots of liquid while the child is learning.

An easy way to teach a child to drink from a straw is to use a cardboard juice container with a straw. Squeeze the container and the juice will move up the straw. Alternatively, you can insert a plastic straw or a piece of aquarium tubing into a plastic ketchup bottle and squeeze the bottle. Aquarium tubing is particulary good for older multihandicapped children.

Throwing eating utensils, especially cups, is a normal phase all children go through. Try to anticipate and catch the hand before the object is thrown. Gently replace it on the table saying, 'That's good. You put it on the table.' You will not always be quick enough. On these occasions, pick up the object calmly with no comment. A lack of a reaction from you lessens the chance of the behaviour being repeated.

Try to make mealtimes pleasant. Include the visually impaired child in family meals whenever possible. The interaction around the table is important to the child's social development. As your child matures and sits at the table with the family, make him aware that food is served from serving dishes on the table. Encourage him to help himself and to be ready to pass the dishes to other people. Show him how to use a knife and fork. He will need lots of practice. Given the opportunity, he can become as skilled as his sighted brothers and sisters. He should be expected to conform to family expectations regarding table manners. If your visually impaired child sometimes participates in setting the table and putting out the food, it helps him to know what tableware is always used and what dishes or utensils are specific to that meal. At the beginning of every meal, tell the family what the meal consists of. Expect the visually impaired child to help clear the table and wash the dishes occasionally.

Dressing and Undressing

While your child is still an infant, as you dress and undress him, form the habit of identifying his body parts. Name the articles of clothing as you put them on and take them off.

When you buy clothing for your child, consider if it will be easy for the child to take it off and put it on. Shoes with Velcro fastenings, pullover tops, pants with elastic waistbands, and loose-fitting clothing will make dressing and undressing easier and more manageable for the child.

Small children frequently take off their socks, shoes, mitts, and hats. To encourage them to take off other garments, pull the garment partway off so that the child needs to give only one pull to get it off. Gradually you do less and less. When you know he is able to undress, he may need an incentive. If he enjoys baths, that would be a good incentive for him to undress. Discourage your child from throwing or dropping his clothes as he takes them off. Until he is old enough to take them to the laundry basket, suggest to him that he place all his clothes in a special spot, e.g., beside his knee on the floor or chair.

Putting on clothes takes much more practice. Dressing and undressing should only be done at the normal routine times of the day, but you will need extra time. Do not do it just as a task in itself. Start with the simple – putting on shoes, pulling pants up the last few inches, or pulling shirts down over the head. When your child reaches

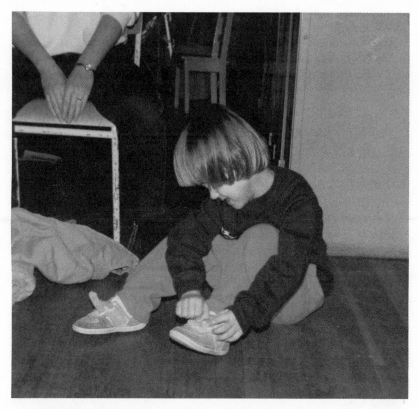

'This time I've got it right!'

this stage, you will need to spend time showing him how to get his arms and legs into clothing. Encourage and challenge him, but do not let him become frustrated. If he has made a good effort, offer to help him. When teaching your child to dress, it is usually easier to stand or sit behind him and work from the back. A small sturdy stool for the child to sit on can sometimes be helpful.

You can help your child find the top or bottom, front or back of a garment by putting a large safety-pin in a predetermined position, and can attach a piece of tape to one shoe to indicate right or left. Opening and closing fastenings come later. Sometimes it helps the child to practise fastening buttons on other family members' clothing. There are no easy ways – it takes time and practice. When you know he is close to being able to dress independently, or he can do it but he takes too long, he may need an incentive, such as an activity that he likes. If he enjoys a ride in the car, you can expect him to make the extra effort to put his clothes on.

Do not be surprised if your child resists wearing a hat or mitts. He uses his ears and hands to tune in to the world. One method of keeping hands warm is to use a muff, so that the child can put his hands in and out as he chooses. Another way is to attach mittens to a string, thread them through the sleeves of his coat, and attach the string at the neck. You can now encourage the child to keep one mitt on at a time without losing the other. Some parents have had success by cutting off the top part of the fingers of a pair of gloves and having the child wear them under the mitts. The hand that is free of a mitt has some protection. You will have to experiment to find the type of hat that is most comfortable for your child. You can try the toque-type hat that can be worn to the tip of the ears or pulled down to cover the ears.

Toilet-training

Toilet-training is a normal process and can be dealt with in the same manner as you would for a sighted child. The child is ready for toilet-training when:

- he is in good health at the time of training
- he is able to retain urine for a fairly long interval between wetting (1–2 hours)
- he has only one or two bowel movements a day
- he shows in some way that he feels ready to urinate or have a bowel movement
- he shows discomfort when soiled or wet

It is easier to start toilet-training in the summer when there are fewer clothes to deal with. Dress the child in clothing that is easy to get on and off, without straps, buttons, or belts. Toilet-training should be treated in a matter-of-fact way. Genuine approval may be given, but avoid undue praise or pressure to perform. Arrange a regular schedule for using the toilet – one that is most likely to catch the child at the time he usually wets or has a bowel movement. Being able to let go requires a lot of practice in timing. For a while he may wet just as he is removed from the toilet seat, or just when he is freshly diapered. *This is a necessary part of the learning* – when to relax at the right moment.

The child needs to feel secure on the toilet seat or potty. Toilet inserts are available. Sit the child on the toilet with his feet firmly supported on a box or stool and with something to hold on to if necessary. If using a potty, place it beside a wall or in a corner and keep it in the same place, preferably in the bathroom. Do not leave the child on the toilet or potty for longer than five or ten minutes or he may forget why he is there. Small boys can learn early to urinate standing up. Place the potty on a stool at the right height for the penis to touch the rim of the potty. Older boys can use the toilet.

Toilet-training hints from parents and teachers:
- One tablespoon of tea ten minutes before taking the child to the toilet increases chances of success and making the point. However, do not use on a regular basis.
- To help locate the toilet bowl, outline the inside edge of the toilet with black tape to provide contrast, or use tin foil tape that reflects the light.
- Have the child urinate in a bucket (sound is encouragement).
- For a good position for older boys, have the child lean over and hold onto the water tank.

For a child who is having unusual difficulty with toilet-training, see further suggestions listed in the case example of Janet at the end of the book.

Sleeping

During the preschool years, all children will occasionally have sleep disturbances. This is normal. Overexcitement, sickness, changes in diet or routine, fears, hospitalization, visitors, new experiences, or even routine visits to a dentist, doctor, etc., can all affect sleep patterns. For the sighted child, the contrast between night and day will usually help in overcoming the problem. For visually impaired children, day and night are less easily defined, and for blind children, night and day can sometimes become reversed. When this happens, it is a difficult problem to overcome.

Whenever possible, prevention is better than cure. A regular routine, fresh air, and exercise are necessary factors in training the child's inner clock and establishing appropriate sleep patterns. For physical and neurological development, a child needs his full quota of undisturbed night's sleep. Sometimes the child's sleeping period can be rearranged to fit into the family's schedule; for example, when the parents are both working, spending time with their child may only be possible in the evening. Parents and children need time together. However, they should understand that a prolonged nap in the day may not obviate the need for a full undisturbed night's sleep, and they ought to adjust their schedules accordingly. On the weekends, do not make significant changes from your established weekday routine.

Some visually impaired children seem to need less sleep than sighted children, perhaps because they are less active. Conversely, there are visually impaired children who sleep too much. Without visual motivation a child may lack interest in his world and may resort to sleep. Personality plays a part. A passive child will need more stimulation to prevent this from happening.

When regular sleep patterns become disturbed, think it through. The difficulty may be traced to one of the problems mentioned earlier. Deal with the situation and then re-establish regular sleep patterns as quickly as possible. At times a child will wake in the night for no apparent reason. Occasionally this happens on several consecutive nights. The child may be too hot, or may be having a recurring dream, not necessarily a bad one. It may be as simple as rolling over too close to the side of the crib and touching the rails. The sighted child may wake up, whimper for a few moments, and because darkness prevents visual stimulation, roll over and fall back to sleep.

For the visually impaired child, darkness may make little difference. He wakes and, as he does in the daytime, finds an interesting activity, and the movement or sound becomes interesting. A common behaviour is bumping the crib back and forth, or bouncing up and down. This quickly brings results. The family wakes up and he receives attention. A few nights of this and his inner clock has been reset!

As you think of a solution, remember the nonvisual perspective. The remedy may need to take into account the visually impaired child's interests, which may be different from those of the sighted child.

Henry's parents stopped him from bumping his crib by tying the crib to a chest of drawers. This stopped the bumping, but did not fully correct the problem. Henry couldn't bump his bed, but he enjoyed the squeak it now made. The squeak kept Henry amused and his family awake. After two wakeful nights, Henry's father dismantled the crib and oiled every movable part that could possibly squeak! It worked. The next night Henry's rocking achieved nothing and he cried loudly. Wisely, his parents did not go to him. After about ten minutes, Henry's crying stopped. His parents heard him singing softly to himself. Then all was quiet. Henry had fallen asleep.

Another youngster, Phyllis, found bouncing in her crib a great night-time sport! Her parents felt they had tried everything and despaired of having a good night's sleep. In frustration, Phyllis's mother tied a sheet over the crib. When Phyllis bounced, her head touched the sheet. She was surprised and tried again with the same result. Phyllis stopped bouncing and, like Henry, wailed her disapproval. Her parents waited anxiously, fearful she would not stop. Phyllis cried for some time and finally fell asleep. This happened for two more nights. Knowing there was nothing seriously wrong, Phyllis's parents let her cry. On the third night Phyllis awoke, whimpered for a few moments, then turned over and went to sleep. A regular sleep routine was once more established.

Another problem can be the blind child who wanders around at night. Parents have found various ways of dealing with this.

Don's father put two peep-holes in the bedroom door. A low light left on in Don's room at night and peep-holes at two different places in the door made it possible to see into the whole room. Don had not mastered opening his bedroom door, and now, even with the door closed, his parents could check on him.

Don was not perturbed by the closed door. He wandered happily around his room. On two occasions he fell asleep on the floor. As he wore sleepers and his room was warm and carpeted, this was not a problem. His parents lifted him back into bed. His mother hung a few items over his bed at a height that he could reach. This increased his interest in staying in bed. It wasn't long before he was sleeping through the night.

There are times when even the most creative solutions do not work. In such cases parents should seek the help of their family doctor. If there is no medical problem, the doctor will probably prescribe a mild sedative that the child can take for a few nights. This will calm the child and enable his parents to reset his inner clock through routine to a normal sleeping pattern. Here is a suggested routine:

a Late afternoon/early evening is time for family frolics. This should be a relaxed time when some excess energy is expended, which is important for the visually impaired child. Aim for a happy time of laughter and sharing. Instead of picking up the evening paper on the way home from work, one father took his two small children, one in the stroller and the other trotting beside him, to the corner store. They bought a paper and two balloons every day!

b Ten minutes before the actual bedtime preparation starts, give a clear warning that it's almost bedtime. Mean it and follow through.

c Baths are warm and relaxing and usually a favourite activity for visually impaired children. Enjoy this time. As you dry your child, start the calming down process: consciously lower your voice a little; slow your movements down; sing songs softly. These details make a tremendous difference – they act like dimming a light.

d A short story or a quiet chat, preferably in the child's room, is an enjoyable part of the bedtime routine. For partially sighted children dim the lights or use a reading-lamp. A small warm drink at this time is helpful. Use a mug with a lid (car travel mugs work well) or a bottle. Finish your story and, while still discussing it, take the child to the toilet. Anticipate all his needs – have his bedtime toy ready, etc.

e Finally, tell him you love him, give him a hug, tuck him in, give him a final kiss, and tell him that you will not be getting him out of bed until morning. Mean it and follow through. Be very consistent. Say what you mean and do it. Little children, whether visually impaired or sighted, are quick to pick up on the inconsistencies of parents. If they know you will come back if they cry a little harder or whine a little longer, they will try. If your child learns early that you mean what you say, he will trust you more and test you less often. This in turn makes it easier for you. Your child will be calmer and you will recognize immediately when something is really wrong. Consistency is a two-way channel. It works for both you and your child.

Here is a technique that works if you have the ability to remain calm in a difficult situation. If this is started from the beginning, it is very easy. It has been used with many preschool and older children, including disturbed foster children.

After you have said good night to your child, you can either close the door or leave it open. This will depend on where the bedroom is situated. If there are bright lights or excessive noise, close the door. If not, leave it open. About three to five minutes after you have said your final good night, go back near your child's room and perform some simple task, close enough so that he can hear you and, if possible, see you. Perhaps you could fold and put away some linen, fetch something from your bedroom, clean the bathroom – anything that takes just a moment or two. Go away again, and repeat a short time later. Do this even if the child appears to be asleep. Occasionally, you might even go into his room, perhaps to return a toy, just for a moment before going out again. Don't hover. Be calm and use a matter-of-fact approach. Do what you were going to do and then leave even if, on seeing or hearing you, your child immediately jumps up and wants attention or screams in rage when you move away. This method is particularly useful if the child is crying when you say your final good night, and is still crying when you perform your tasks or go into his room. Do not start *any* conversation, even if he's screaming. Do not try to lay him down or cover him up. As you go out, leaving the door as it had been, you might say, 'I love you. See you in the morning.' That's all. No conversation. Say it in a calm, normal voice. Do not speak louder so that he can hear – preferably softer. If he wants to hear you, he'll have to quiet down! *Act as if your child is behaving perfectly normally*, and give no indication that his behaviour bothers you. For a child who is used to getting attention by screaming or using other persuasive means – e.g., 'Need to pee pee,' 'Want a drink,' 'Want to see Daddy,' 'Want to go back to my Mummy' – it can take two or three nights. Felicity has found that it has never taken longer than a week. A few nights of bedtime fuss is better than months of night-time nonsense!

This technique works because it gives the child a sense of security. He learns that his parent loves him; that she means what she says and his screaming, crying, and pleading do not work; that his parent is close by and life goes on as usual even when he sleeps; that noise and threats do not intimidate. If you can give this clear message to your child early in life, night-time routines can become a pleasure. This method also helps to get him accustomed to your presence as he settles down to sleep, so that he will not be anxious if you ever need to be nearby out of concern.

Toys

Toys are a part of a child's daily life. Parents of visually impaired children frequently find that toys do not interest their children. This is usually because the visually impaired child is not attracted by the toy's visual appeal. He does not see the possibilities for play, nor does he understand the toy's representative factor.

When introducing a toy to a visually impaired child, it is helpful first to separate in your own mind the various aspects of the toy – the pieces, colour, shape, contours, texture, moving parts, sound, smell, etc. Now focus on one aspect. If the toy has several pieces, put away all but one and let the child play with that one piece. This helps him become aware and familiar with that piece, its shape, size, and properties. Do the same with the other pieces and finally bring them all together. If a sound-maker is part of the toy, do not automatically start with that. This is often used best as the climax after you have found creative and fun ways to use the separate pieces, e.g., roll the pieces, hide them in the child's clothing or in an adult's pockets, thread them, play with them in water if appropriate, blow into them or put them into containers.

When you present a simple toy to an infant, you have an opportunity to learn more about the infant by observing how he responds to it. Is the colour, texture, or sound attracting his attention or making him avoid the toy? Does he examine it with any part of his body (hand, foot, face, tongue) or turn his head in a particular way? Can he grasp it, bring his hands to the middle of his body, or retrieve it when it drops? Does he shake it against his own body, enjoying the sensation as well as the sound? Does he explore all of the toy? Has he found only the handle? Does he know there is another part? This is another way of tuning in to your child.

STEPS TO INDEPENDENCE

'Me do it,' demands a young child, much to the frustration of a busy parent. Children learn by imitation. They see other people accomplishing certain tasks, and want to imitate. The visually impaired child is less likely to ask to do something on his own, as he cannot see how other people operate. After working hard to teach a young visually impaired child a skill such as dressing, parents and teachers frequently complain that the child is lazy or stubborn because he refuses to perform the task without their help. Usually this is neither stubbornness nor laziness, but what might be termed 'learned helplessness.' During the teaching process the child has performed on cues of touch or voice, and is not aware that his parent's or teacher's goal is to help him perform the task independently. He has not seen other people put on clothes without help, so does not understand that this is what he is expected to do. During the teaching process, the parent or teacher gives the child praise and encouragement, then knowing he is capable of doing the task, they stop prompting and may become irritated at the child's seeming lack of cooperation. This is confusing for the child because from his perception, the situation has not changed. He waits for the same cues of touch or voice as he had before, and cannot understand the change in the adult's attitude. Although the child may have been told and encouraged to do the task independently, he may not have reached the cognitive level of understanding himself as an autonomous being. He understands the direction and encouragement only as further prompting towards his perceived role as an extension of the adult. This confusion is more apparent if the child is blind. However, partially sighted children also experience confusion.

Partially sighted children's eye conditions can be very difficult to understand for those who are sighted. A partially sighted child may be observed running freely around a familiar environment, appearing to function as if he were fully sighted. In reality his distance vision may only allow him to see objects as shadows or hazy blobs of colours or movement. This same child, with his face close to the book, may be able to pick out tiny details on a page without seeing the total picture. An observer may find it difficult to comprehend that the child does not have a clear understanding of what is going on around him. Like the blind child, a partially sighted child may not have the ability to see others putting on clothes and he too may not understand that he is expected to dress independently. When visual imitation is difficult for a child, the learning process may be slower.

Jessica was a bright two-year-old with limited vision. She had a healthy appetite and enjoyed a variety of foods. In spite of this, mealtimes were frustrating for Jessica and her mother. Jessica persistently resisted her mother's efforts to encourage her to use a spoon independently. The hand-over-hand approach and verbal request that she use her spoon were not working. One evening, tired and frustrated, Jessica's mother complained to her husband. 'Don't worry so,' he said. 'She's bound to be slower. Remember, she can't see very well.' His response added to his wife's frustration. Later it occurred to her that perhaps that was the problem.

At lunch the following day, her mother sat Jessica on her lap and showed her how she used her spoon to eat. Jessica was interested. She tried to help and even attempted to put the spoon in her own mouth. At supper her parents were delighted when she ate four spoonfuls independently.

For the totally blind child, visual imitation will never be possible; therefore, the adult will need to use techniques to assist the blind child. A sighted child has opportunities for observation long before he is expected to perform a task. Tasks will be more easily accomplished by the blind child if he too has the equivalent of an observation period. The following are some suggestions.

Toilet training
• Months before toilet-training begins, introduce the child to the potty and toilet. Allow time for exploration.
• Have the blind child accompany family members when they use toilet facilities.
• Allow the child to become comfortable with sitting on the potty or toilet. Place the potty on your knee and sit the child on it. Remember that this experience is replacing observation and the child is not expected to use the potty – just get used to sitting on it.
• Sit the child on the toilet with his feet firmly supported on a box or stool with something to hold on to if necessary.

Dressing and undressing
• Let the child play games with Dad, pulling his gloves or slippers on and off.
• Sit the child on Mum's knee while she pulls on and buttons up her sweater, and later when she takes it off again.
• Help take someone's hat, boots, etc., off and put them on again.

Mealtimes
• Before the infant is off the bottle, let him experience the feel of a china cup, plastic mug, or glass on his lips.
• Give frequent opportunities to feel food on spoon or dish.
• Help the child become aware of others eating by occasionally allowing him to sit on an adult's lap during mealtimes.

Independence or dependence on self will be increased in a visually impaired child if the adult recognizes and provides the child with experiences that will compensate for his inability to observe and imitate. The principle of exploration to replace observation holds true in all early learning situations.

Relating to Environmental Information

A sighted preschooler can be upstairs, downstairs, out into the yard, over to a neighbour's and back, and all in a very short time. The apartment-dwelling preschooler will be no less adventuresome, trotting from room to room, climbing over and under furniture, turning out drawers and cupboards, and being all too anxious to 'assist' in the daily housekeeping chores.

A visually impaired preschooler may be just as adventurous and require the same amount of activity, yet he may often rock back and forth, reciting TV commercials and other jingles, or repetitiously manipulate a toy. For this preschooler, the potential for interesting and constructive play is not obvious, and consequently spontaneous exploration and 'assisting' happens less frequently.

Sighted children have a panoramic vista of areas for potential exploration and adventure. For the visually impaired child, however, this roving is limited to as far as his body can reach, and intervention is usually required to encourage him to move freely and explore. In this context the visually impaired child who has brothers and sisters, in particular an active younger sibling, may have an advantage. As the younger, sighted child explores, learns, and verbalizes, he becomes a source of information for the visually impaired child, often motivating him towards greater action and exploration.

Just as a visually impaired preschooler will need to be encouraged to explore, the visually impaired infant will also need to be made aware of his environment and shown how to reach out and explore it. To some parents, making the child aware of his surroundings is so natural that they are not consciously aware they are interacting. When the infant doesn't reach out for Daddy's beard, Daddy takes the little hand to explore the beard. The small hands are encouraged to search for Mother's hair, necklace, earrings, or bracelet, to find the bottle or cookie. The infant is placed in a sitting, crawling, or standing position and then encouraged to move his whole body to the enthusiastic promptings of his parents or caregivers.

For other equally caring parents or caregivers, such interaction isn't such a natural or easy occurrence. Their personalities are different. They need feedback that the sighted infant gives – the reaching out,

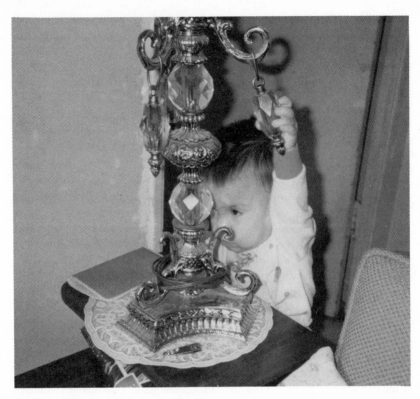

'There's something above my head!'

the smile of recognition, the eye contact, and visual interaction. Spontaneous chatter is not easy for them. The visually impaired infant's seeming lack of response is disturbing or interpreted as contentment and they will rejoice at having a 'good, easy baby.'

It is vision that encourages a baby to lift his head, to reach out or to crawl forward, to take that first faltering step, to examine a toy, and as he matures, to venture out to the spaces beyond, to run, to climb, and to explore. Without vision or with limited vision, directed help and encouragement must be given to allow the infant or child to follow the same, natural developmental steps as his sighted contemporary.

The secret of making interaction work is to ensure that it has a purpose from the infant's or child's perspective. An infant lifts his head to see something nearby or to be closer to his parents. The preschooler reaches for the cookie because he sees it there and knows it tastes good! The visually impaired child must be helped to understand why it is worth his while to reach out and move forward. Parents and caregivers, especially those for whom spontaneous chatter is an effort, will find interaction much easier and often more valuable if they try to have the child close to them whenever possible. If the infant or child is close by when the dishes are washed, it is very easy to say, 'Smell the dishwashing soap,' or 'Feel the sugar Mummy has spilled on your tray.' For the older preschooler it might be, 'I'll lift you up so that you can get the jam from the high shelf,' or 'Shall we see if we can find the cold eggs and milk in the fridge?' If the child is left in the play-pen, crib, or another room, this interaction is less likely to happen.

One preschooler looked forward to bedmaking time because she was 'hidden' in the bed and tickled through the blankets before each bed was made, and then was allowed 'three very little bounces' on the now smooth, freshly made bed. She also liked it when her mother put her feet into her father's big, furry slippers and they shuffled to the closet to put them away. When she was older, she found her mother's high-heel shoes in the closet and also a variety of interesting purses and belts. But the interest began with her father's slippers, long before she could even walk!

Another mother carried her infant in a back sling when she did the vacuuming. When he became older and heavier, she gave him occasional rides on the noisy vacuum cleaner and taught him how he could turn off the noise and turn it on again. Before he went to nursery school, he'd felt the suction of the vacuum, been shown how a piece of paper was suctioned up, and then shown how the canister could be opened and the paper found inside. He understood the vacuum noise and was therefore not afraid of it. Whenever possible, sounds should be given meaning.

Visually impaired children may hear a sound in the distance, but unless it is related to their understanding of something they have physically explored, it will have very little meaning to them. Tell the child, 'That's a bird,' or even be more specific and say, 'That's a cardinal' or 'woodpecker,' so that the child will have a name for the sound of a bird. Teach the child names for sounds. One blind child took great pleasure in the many bird sounds he could accurately identify. It is, however, very important that a sound be connected to a substance and a reality that the child can understand. It is not difficult to find a bird for the child to experience. Pet shops and zoos, if the need is explained, are often most willing to help. On a farm there are usually chickens and ducks that can be touched. When a child has experienced a real bird, stuffed birds or models can be helpful in furthering the child's understanding.

Detailed descriptions are not always necessary, but it is important that a sound is not left as an abstract to confuse the child later. Vision identifies sounds, but even common sounds can be confusing to the visually impaired child. One preschool blind child called frantically to his father to get the oilcan to stop the squeak. The 'squeak' was the cry of seagulls.

> For some years one totally blind child could identify the sound of the blender. 'That's the blender,' Laurie would say, although she had no idea what a blender was. One day she was shown a blender. This caused Laurie to become very upset and even a little angry. Presumably she had formed her own fanciful idea of what the sound represented. After several experiences of helping to put the food into the blender, feeling the vibrations when it was turned on, and then feeling the processed food, she exchanged her fanciful idea for reality. After this experience, whenever she said, 'That's the blender,' there was an air of satisfaction in her voice.

Daily activities around the home help a sighted child to anticipate events – for example, the sun coming through the curtains or the light going on in the next bedroom; the toilet flushing; the sound of Dad shaving; the clatter of dishes downstairs; the kettle whistling; the coffee percolating or the smell of cooking; the shower upstairs; the dog being let out and the cat fed. These are all morning activities. Later, there may be a short, quiet time. The older children have gone to school and Dad to work. Mother may sip coffee and briefly glance at the newspaper. Then the morning routines begin. One day the routine is changed. The shopping cart is pulled out indicating that it's time for the weekly shopping expedition. Throughout the day and week, there are clues to the comings and goings of the household. Smell, hearing, and vision all play a part in identifying different times of the day, but it is vision that confirms them.

For the visually impaired child, in particular the blind child, these clues are very important, but they can only be fully utilized if they have been identified and, whenever possible, experienced a few times for confirmation. A father could let his visually impaired daughter feel his rough face before shaving, allow her to listen to the noise of the shaver, and then feel his stubble-free face. The shaving-cream can be identified, felt, and smelled. If this is done on a few occasions, the sound of the shaver will then be meaningful. Once in a while it is helpful for families and teachers of visually impaired infants and children to consciously listen to the sounds around them. This helps the adult to be more aware of what associations the visually impaired child may be making.

A mother had said goodbye to her family and left for work. The four-year-old blind child had heard all this, but asked five minutes later, 'When's Mummy going to work?' The baby-sitter said, 'You know Mummy's already gone to work.' The child seemed puzzled and repeated her question a few minutes later. The baby-sitter stopped what she was doing, picked up the child, and went to the window. To her astonishment, the car was stopped at the end of the drive and the child's mother was in conversation with a neighbour. The baby-sitter was puzzled. The next day the curious baby-sitter asked the child to tell her when her mother had gone to work. She held the child and watched out of the window. 'She's gone now, she's on the road,' the child said. The child had been listening for the sound of the engine as the car turned onto the road! For her, that was the point when Mummy had gone to work. Saying goodbye was only preparation for going.

Identifying sounds and smells can prove to be very important, as one mother found out when her blind child told her the fridge was broken. He had not heard the usual turning on and off of the motor during the day, the sounds of which his mother was seldom aware. Sighted people may not be aware of sounds in the same way as a blind person. Making young, visually impaired children aware of sounds, smells, and tastes and identifying them is another way of helping them to effectively interact with their environment. Accurate identification will also facilitate language development, as it is not primarily vision but sounds, smells, tastes, and touch on which the visually impaired child's communication is based.

All small children enjoy music. However, when the child is visually impaired, parents and teachers tend to use it too much to occupy the child and keep him content and quiet. While this is sometimes necessary, constant background music may prevent the visually impaired child from picking up some valuable information about his environment.

Many people become very upset because they believe there is so much they cannot explain to a visually impaired child. This can be another form of the feeling of loss. It may also be the frustration of not knowing how to explain, or the sadness of not being able to share a particular experience. Most experiences that can be explained to a sighted child can be explained to a blind child, providing visual terms are avoided.

> Rob was swinging a toy. His mother said, 'You'd better be careful or you'll break the mirror.' 'What's a mirror?' the child asked. 'That big piece of glass right beside you,' his mother replied. 'What's it for?' he asked, feeling it. 'Can I shake it? Does it make a noise?' To each negative response he became more insistent. When it is difficult to know how to answer, a question will often help or give a clue. His mother asked, 'How do you know or learn about something?' Rob hesitated for a moment and then said, 'I feel it with my fingers or I ask somebody.' 'Well, a mirror is something like that, but it only works for people who use their eyes to tell them about things. I can be your mirror. If you come to me with your coat and hat on, I can tell you if the buttons are done up or if your hat is on straight,' his mother explained. 'I can do that myself,' Rob said. 'Then I guess you don't need a mirror.' Rob laughed and ran off to play. He had never experienced seeing, so it didn't mean anything to him.

A visually impaired child gains independence or dependency on self when he can relate to and act on environmental information. For him, this takes longer and requires more energy and thought on the part of the sighted caregiver. It is also very rewarding to observe the child's budding awareness of the world around him and to know that even visual experiences can be shared and enjoyed together.

Problem Solving

People must have basic information if they are to solve problems. This is especially true for the visually impaired child. As emphasized in this book, sighted people can obtain information at a glance, but may forget that the most basic information they have received so quickly, and often incidentally, may be unavailable to a blind person.

Problem solving begins early in life. Parents of a blind infant are frequently disappointed and also confused when the infant does not reach out or crawl towards the musical toy placed near him. When they see their friend's infant, sometimes younger than their own child, who is reaching out and crawling, they may become alarmed.

Fearing that blindness is not their child's only disability, they cannot think clearly and recognize a simple fact. The visually impaired child may not know that the pleasing noise he is listening to is part of a toy that he might also enjoy touching! This is very basic information that the sighted infant learns instantly through vision. If the sighted child had not perceived the sound to be part of the toy, he too might not have made the extra effort to move forward.

The *object permanence* factor – knowing that something is still there even though it cannot be seen – is also involved in problem solving. In the latter half of their first year, sighted infants usually begin to understand that although objects may be out of view, they are still there. When a sighted child is developing object permanence and sees a cushion fall onto the toy he was just playing with, he begins to understand that the toy may be still under the cushion. Object permanence affects many areas of a blind child's life. Some educators believe that understanding object permanence is one of the major keys to a blind child's development.

What does object permanence have to do with problem solving? Everything! Consider the sighted baby whose toy is covered by a cushion. If the baby does not know the toy is still there hidden under the cushion, what reason does he have to pull that cushion out of the way? Information motivates the child to problem solve. When information is inadequate, the visually impaired child's efforts to solve problems are hampered.

Five-year-old Erica helped her mother make their lunch every day. A favourite was peanut butter. They had it often, stuffed into celery sticks, rolled in lettuce or in a sandwich with jam, honey, or bacon. Sometimes, for a special treat, they made peanut butter balls. The routine was for Erica's mother to put all the items on the table. Erica had become very proficient and seldom needed help. One day, Erica's mother forgot the peanut butter. Erica looked closely and then felt around the table. 'The peanut butter is not here,' she said in surprise. 'Oh, that's right. I forgot to take it out of the cupboard,' her mother said. At that moment the doorbell rang. While her mother was answering the door, Erica considered the kitchen. There was the broom closet into which she helped her mother put the vacuum. There was the small cupboard in which her mother kept the Tupperware. There were the fridge, the dishwasher, and the drawers for kitchen utensils. Then she remembered the closet where the cookie sheets were kept. That's where it must be, she thought, on the other side of the cookie sheets. When her mother returned, she was astonished to find Erica feeling around in the back of the cupboard.

'I can't find the peanut butter,' Erica said. In a flash Erica's mother realized Erica could not see enough to know that there were cupboards above the counter and it had never occurred to her to show Erica. She showed them to Erica immediately. Thereafter Erica helped put everything away after shopping expeditions. Her parents decided that Erica would learn where everything belonged in the house. In time Erica learned about the kitchen, bathroom, her father's workshop, the garden tool-shed, and much more. She also learned to problem solve. For example, she found that she could climb onto the counter and reach the highest shelf in the kitchen with the help of a chair. Erica delighted in her ever-expanding world.

As described earlier, information motivates a child, even an infant, to explore further. We often think of it the other way around: motivation as the gateway to information. Of course this is also true. A child will not be motivated to explore without information, and without motivation he will not explore and gain more information. Everything is interdependent. Forgetting this interdependency is one of the main reasons why sighted people often experience difficulty in meeting the need of a blind child. The problem stems from a one-sided approach. Instead of asking, 'What can I do to motivate him?' you may find the solution more easily if you think it through from a different angle, asking yourself, 'What information does the child need to have in order to be motivated?' When trying to find a solution, it is important to think clearly about whose problem it is we are trying to solve – our own or the child's. If both, then our solution must solve both. Never forget interdependency; each factor depends on another.

Martin was blind. His teacher wanted him to move independently around the nursery school. Unless led, Martin always remained in the place he was left, never venturing to explore on his own. Finally, one teacher discovered a method that worked. She gave Martin a music box, which Martin enjoyed. The teacher then took it from him and placed it a short distance away and suggested that Martin find it. To her delight, Martin moved forward very quickly and picked up the music box. He was warmly congratulated. After a few days, Martin could go from one room to the other to find the music box. The problem was solved, or was it? But whose problem was solved? The teacher's problem was temporarily solved, but Martin's hadn't even been addressed. Instead of being led by the teacher, he was now being led by the music box!

When the teacher took Martin's hand, he had no choice but to move because he was being led. When he followed the music box, he could decide not to seek the source of the music and, in fact, after two weeks he did just that. He decided this game was no longer fun. The music box was no more interesting than the other sounds around him, which he preferred to listen to while he rocked and flapped his hands. What was even more distressing for the teachers was that Martin now resisted all musical toys. When someone showed him one, he wanted no part of it. If they took his hand to explore it, Martin became angry. Now he not only did not want to move around, but he was considered tactile defensive.

The teachers decided they would forget about encouraging him to move around. They would concentrate instead on what he most enjoyed and build information about that. They started with the indoor slide by showing him as much as they could about it. He learned to slide down holding on and not holding on. He went down on his tummy and on his back; feet first and even head first. He was also allowed to walk up the slide and down the slide, just for the experience. He learned that there were only certain ways that the slide should be used. He was shown why it was dangerous to walk up and down the slide or to come down head first. He was not just told, he was shown. For a whole week, Martin played on the slide and had fun. The teachers were rewarded by his laughter. His hand flapping was less, but he still needed to be led around. The next week he learned words for body positions like 'keep your heels on the slide,' or 'bend your knees,' or 'land on your toes.'

Each day Martin learned something new and was always given time to practise on the things he understood. The teachers concentrated on making all learning experiences enjoyable. The more fun Martin had, the more he learned. As Martin gained experiences, he was given simple responsibilities. He was asked to show Susie how to go down the slide on her tummy. He learned to wait while others had their turns on the slide. The slide and other play equipment became the motivators. By the end of the year, Martin moved freely in the nursery school. He now helped give out cookies, went to the washroom on his own, and began to interact with the other children. A visitor to the school was amazed to learn that Martin was blind!

The teachers had found a major problem solver. Start with what the child most enjoys and is familiar with and build information on that. Knowing and using what the child enjoys is important, but there is another aspect of this also. The child must know what is expected of him and see a purpose for it from his perspective. This is an ongoing process. If the purpose becomes obsolete, it loses its effectiveness.

Initially, the purpose from Martin's point of view was to find the music box. It lost its effectiveness when Martin became bored with what he had perceived to be a game. He did not understand that the teacher's expectation was for him to move around the room. If the teacher had realized in time, she could have turned the game into a motivator to encourage him to move and to increase his familiarity with the room. She might have said, 'I'm putting the music box on the slide. Listen for the music. Can you find the slide?' Martin could have been given a few minutes to play with the music box and then shown some fun things to do on the slide. Each of the other areas in the nursery school could have been found and explored in the same way.

We have been discussing problem solving in relation to information and motivation. Another aspect of problem solving that children need to be introduced to early is that of correcting mistakes. Parents and teachers can use the mistakes that they themselves make as learning experiences for the child. For example, they can exclaim and tell the child what has happened. This part often occurs quite automatically. However, the next step is usually forgotten. The child needs to be told what the adult is going to do to correct the mistake. For example, if something has been broken, the child can be told that there are pieces all over the floor and that these pieces need to be swept up. He then needs to be shown the pieces and learn how they can cut and hurt people. He also needs to know whether the pieces are put in the indoor garbage or the outside garbage. They could then discuss how the broken object will be replaced, if replacing it is possible, and if not, why not. Learning that some things are easily replaced and others are more precious is also important.

The child also needs to understand that even adults can become upset. Sighted children, even small ones, can see by their parents' expression that their parents are unhappy. The visually impaired child may not be aware of this fact. He too needs to know these details. It helps him to understand himself and others. When the mistake is the child's – for example when he knocks over his juice – it can also be a learning experience. However, too much teaching can cause tension. If the child has already learned from a similar experience, it will be easier. If not, it is better not to force the child through the whole process of cleaning up, but rather emphasize only key points. The glass is empty. His sandwich, chair, and floor are wet. These he can feel and experience. After everything is cleaned up, the difference can be pointed out. 'Feel how dry your tray is now and hold the glass while I pour more juice in.' All children spill, break, and make other mistakes many times. The steps to correcting these mistakes can be an ongoing process. As the child learns that he and others make mistakes, it is easier to help him work through his and know how to find the solutions. It should be remembered that similar attention is required for less concrete mistakes, such as an incorrectly phrased sentence, inappropriate directions, getting lost, putting on the wrong clothes, hurting someone's feelings.

> Marjorie was totally blind. On her sixth birthday, Mrs West, who lived next door, gave her a Barbie doll. Mrs West's daughter loved playing with dolls and she thought Marjorie would enjoy it too. However, Marjorie took no interest in the doll and had to be pressured to say thank you.
>
> Later, Marjorie's mother talked to her and explained that Mrs West's feelings had been hurt. 'She was very sad. Sometimes your feelings are hurt. Remember that time John told you to go away? I think Mrs West felt like you did then. It was disappointing for you to get a Barbie doll, but it was kind of Mrs West to remember your birthday, wasn't it?' 'Yes,' replied Marjorie. 'Next time you will know to say thank you,' her mother said gently.

Problems must be correctly identified. For the visually impaired child, independence or dependency on self can be achieved when he has the appropriate information to enable him to solve problems and correct mistakes.

Challenging Opportunities

As in all aspects of life, judgment and balance are necessary. Not all challenges are positive and what may be expedient for one person may be totally inappropriate for another. However, challenge is as much a part of life as growing and developing. In fact, it can be seen as an integral part of both. Without challenge both intellectual and physical growth may be impeded and one's potential not realized. Challenges are not peculiar to any age or state, rich or poor. From infancy through old age, they can goad and motivate one to a fuller and more rewarding life.

Challenge in one form or another is a daily occurrence for youngsters and a necessary part of growing up. Challenges may be self-imposed or provided by competition and games of many kinds. Something more is learned about oneself with each challenge. A timid or immature child may need encouragement to accept a new and simple challenge, while a more adventurous youngster may need to be held back and encouraged or taught to think constructively before acting. Each child, regardless of his ability, should have the opportunity to experience and learn through challenge.

The visually impaired child may not be aware of the opportunities available to him. As he is unable to see the total scenario, he will have difficulty in judging the situation and will need an adult to assist him. It may be necessary to explain or show him what needs to be done and then encourage him to do it. Others' accomplishments will also need to be explained to the visually impaired child. Like his peers, he should have the chance to emulate a hero – this can be his father, a friend, or a well-known personality.

A challenge should not be a chore but something that adds to the joy of living. It will be a struggle that yields satisfaction.

Amos was blind and attended a regular kindergarten in his community. In some areas Amos was delayed and a special teacher had been hired to help him catch up. A minor difficulty Amos had was learning how to pull on his boots. Finally, through the persistence and help of his special teacher, he learned to do it. Now Amos, like most of the other children, could put on his boots independently. There was no particular satisfaction for Amos in it; it was just a daily chore that had to be done and Amos did it. One day his mother arrived early to take him on an outing. Amos had pulled on one boot and was starting on the other when, to his pleasure, his mother arrived, greeted him, and pulled the other boot on for him. The teacher interrupted sharply, 'You didn't have to do that, you know. He's quite capable of doing it himself.'

Startled, Amos's mother said, 'Oh yes, I know he can do it. Since coming to school he does it every morning when I am getting the baby ready. I'm sorry.' The special teacher said no more and moved away. The happy interaction between mother and son had been interrupted. There was an air of tension.

Very often disabled children are put into the position of proving themselves, not for their own satisfaction, but for the satisfaction of those who have struggled to teach them. It is an easy trap for parents and teachers to fall into. Amos had already acquired the skill of putting on his boots. Although a visually impaired child may need more practice than his sighted peers, there is no reason why he should not have help occasionally. Sighted children are also given help from time to time. Children should experience the pleasure of being helped, which is the beginning of learning to be helpful to others.

A skill can be used as a challenge: 'Amos, Daddy will be home at any moment. Surprise him and get your boots on before he comes in the door. Then you'll be ready to go shopping with him. Listen, I can hear the car coming.' Amos then has an opportunity to choose whether or not he will accept the challenge. If the child has not constantly been made to prove himself, he will probably accept willingly and enjoy the fun.

Those who work hard to teach a skill to a child with special difficulties do not always recognize how hard the child has already worked, or that in accomplishing the task he has put in far more effort than other children. However small the child's accomplishments, it is important for parents, teachers, and the child to feel a sense of pride and satisfaction. However, care should be taken to ensure that the child is not pressured to perform unnecessarily.

It is unlikely that anyone would knowingly deprive a visually impaired child of an opportunity, yet it is often those who are the most caring and concerned for the child's well-being who do the depriving! This form of deprivation has many labels: overprotection, pity, overindulgence, love, fear, overwork, lack of time, and lack of understanding. It may not be conscious or deliberate, but it is deprivation just the same. Allowing the child to have the opportunity of an extra challenge is not always easy, especially for those who care the most. However, these challenges allow the child to prove himself and add to the joy of living.

When helping a child achieve independence, the challenge is sometimes more the parent's than the child's. Some infants, particularly those with a passive personality, will be quite content to stay in one position or place, and may protest loudly if not permitted to do so.

Rhoda, totally blind, was one of these infants. She was a beautiful baby, happy and responsive, but she had no wish to move! If she was given a toy, Rhoda shook it happily. If she dropped it and felt where it fell, she would pick it up. If not, she would shake her hands and head and remain gurgling happily to herself. Rhoda had learned to sit when she was seven months old and providing she heard people around her and had her daily needs of food and drink met, she remained happy. Seven months later Rhoda was heavier, but had changed very little. She still sat without moving. When her mother took her hand to help her search for a toy she didn't mind, but if the searching meant she needed to move her whole body, then she objected. If she was placed on her tummy, that was the last straw. She roared her disapproval. Her mother was sure Rhoda must be in pain or frightened and quickly returned her to her sitting position. Immediately Rhoda smiled. But Rhoda was fourteen months old. Rhoda's mother was becoming worried. She had been assuring herself that Rhoda would be slower because she couldn't see and that in her own good time Rhoda would move like other children. Now she was doubting her theory.

One day Rhoda's aunt and ten-month-old cousin came to visit for a week. Todd was fully sighted and he was crawling all over the place, including over Rhoda. When Todd sat on her head, that was too much. Rhoda spluttered, rolled herself over onto her tummy, and felt for Todd. Rhoda's mother couldn't believe what she was seeing and quickly stopped her sister from moving Todd away. That was the moment of realization. Rhoda's mother now knew Rhoda could lie on her tummy and would reach out. She also realized she had a challenge. She had to find a way to make Rhoda want to move.

Rhoda's mother found observing Todd to be a real help. She noticed, for example, how quickly Todd went for his bottle if it rolled away and decided that Rhoda could also be taught to find her bottle. When Rhoda was really hungry, she placed her on the floor on her tummy; of course, Rhoda protested, but her mother took her hand and stretched it out to touch the bottle. Rhoda couldn't quite get hold of it and she was furious. As Rhoda kicked out in anger, her foot touched the table leg. She pushed against it and propelled herself forward. She grabbed the bottle, immediately rolling onto her back to drink. Rhoda's mother and aunt were delighted. Rhoda's aunt suggested that it would be a good idea to put Rhoda's feet close to a wall or heavy object until she understood the idea of moving forward.

When Rhoda was two, her aunt and Todd came to visit again. Rhoda had learned to walk four months earlier. She still wasn't too steady and walked with her legs far apart, but she crawled and bummed her way around very quickly. Rhoda's dad told her aunt, 'Not long after you left, your sister worked hard to teach her to crawl. Finally Rhoda was on her hands and knees, but she just rocked back and forth. She would not move forward. We worked together to show her how to move forward and finally we succeeded. Rhoda would move to either her mother or me. We could not find a way to make Rhoda lift her head up. Try as we would, she insisted on touching her head to the floor when she moved. She would only lift her head up if she was still. We solved the problem. Rhoda loves her bath. One day we filled the bath up a little fuller than usual and put Rhoda on her tummy. Of course Rhoda lifted up her head. Watch,' he said. 'Rhoda, show us how you used to crawl with your head on the floor.' Rhoda did. 'How did you learn to crawl in the bath?' Rhoda immediately lifted up her head. Rhoda's aunt said, 'Rhoda gave you a challenge and you met it. I can hardly believe how she has progressed.'

Like Rhoda, many blind children rock back and forth in the crawl position, but do not move forward. As well as needing the motivation to move, one must realize that in the crawl position it is the head that first comes in contact with an object. Usually the greatest incentive is to move forward to a parent. Independence or dependency on self for the visually impaired child is achieved when problems are not avoided, but seen as opportunities for greater challenge towards new accomplishments and self-awareness.

Learning to Communicate Meaningfully

Language and communication are not the same. Many visually impaired children know words, but not all can communicate. Some can communicate but do not use words. There are two aspects to language – receptive and expressive. Receptive language is the ability to understand and form ideas about what is being said. Expressive language is the ability to verbalize or express your thoughts or ideas. Receptive language always precedes expressive language. Long before a child can speak, receptive language is being developed.

Communication is a complex system learned from infancy through imitation and practice. For many people, it is only when the system breaks down that they think about it. To know how to help the visually impaired child to communicate meaningfully, it is necessary to think through and understand the communication sequence.

The illustration showing cognitive steps to meaningful communication demonstrates that communication is interrelated with concept development. The components of communication are more than knowing the meaning of words and having information. They include all the subtleties of voice inflections, eye contact, facial expression, gesture, stance, plus the many different connotations

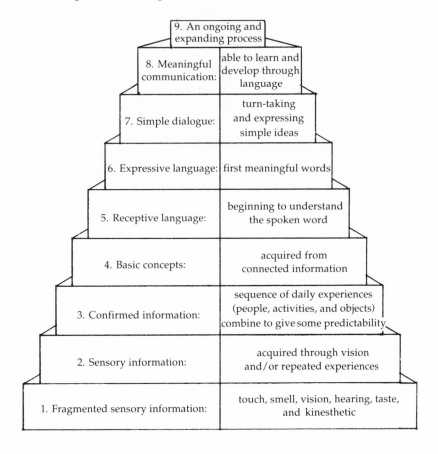

9. An ongoing and expanding process	
8. Meaningful communication:	able to learn and develop through language
7. Simple dialogue:	turn-taking and expressing simple ideas
6. Expressive language:	first meaningful words
5. Receptive language:	beginning to understand the spoken word
4. Basic concepts:	acquired from connected information
3. Confirmed information:	sequence of daily experiences (people, activities, and objects) combine to give some predictability
2. Sensory information:	acquired through vision and/or repeated experiences
1. Fragmented sensory information:	touch, smell, vision, hearing, taste, and kinesthetic

Cognitive Steps to Meaningful Communication

attached to each of these. Communication also involves turn-taking, listening, responding, and initiating. It requires that the person know when to speak, who is being spoken to, when he is being heard, and if what he is saying is being listened to and understood. Hearing and listening are not the same. You may have heard a person speak, but you may not have listened to what he said.

We have mentioned some of the many facets of language and communication and their relationship to concept development. Vision is an integral part of the total communication system.

Language is visual. To make a statement that does not have some visual connotation is difficult. A visually impaired child must learn to speak in a totally visual language. It is necessary to think through and recognize the potential difficulties before they happen. Knowing the cause of problems makes it easier to prevent them and to know what to do if they should arise. A visually impaired child's communication must not be taken for granted. This is especially true if the child has minimal or no vision. As communication affects every area of the child's development, a special effort must be made to help him to understand words and develop communication skills. Communication difficulties experienced by a visually impaired child are often the root cause of seemingly unrelated problems. As communication can only be effective when concepts and connections are accurate, it is an ongoing process. In this section we will discuss what steps can be taken to make communication in a visual language easier for a nonvisual child.

Bond with an infant. Communication starts from day one. Long before words are understood, mother and baby develop a relationship through their own very special communication. This special relationship is referred to as bonding and is an essential part of infant development. Sometimes parents of blind infants experience difficulty in bonding.

> 'I don't think he likes me,' Irene, a young mother, said tearfully. 'He hardly ever responds. The doctor said the test showed he was only blind. Could the doctor be wrong?,' she asked. Piers was four months old. Irene recognized that Piers seemed very unresponsive. He did not smile or gurgle when she spoke to him or picked him up.

Not all parents recognize what is wrong or are able to express it as clearly as Irene did. For most it is a nebulous feeling that they cannot describe. Irene felt rejected by her small son. She fed him and cared for him but did not enjoy him. Their times together became shorter and shorter. Instead of lingering over meal and change times to cuddle and play with him, she put him back into the crib where Piers seemed happiest. Irene was miserable and secretly worried. The problem was a lack of eye contact and facial expression. Instead of smiles and gurgles Piers became quiet and still in anticipation of his mother's special touch. Even at an early age personalities are evident. Some infants are quiet and passive, others active and restless. Some express themselves with facial movements, gurgling, and squirming, while others, like Piers, become still and quiet, their faces almost expressionless.

Be observant of body language.
After the problem had been explained to Irene, she was quick to pick up on Piers's body language. She noticed that if she talked softly to him and stroked his hand he twitched his legs each time she stopped as if to say, 'Why did you stop, Mum?' Irene spent more time with Piers and began to enjoy him, except for one thing. He didn't seem to like being cuddled. He would throw his arms up and pull back. This too was body language. Piers had become used to lying flat on his back in his crib, his arms up. In this position he felt safe, his whole body supported by the mattress. When Irene understood that Piers was telling her he felt insecure with nothing against his back, she would lie on the chesterfield with him resting his back against her body. Irene sang and rocked Piers and played with his hands to bring his arms forward. As soon as Piers was relaxed and happy in this position, she turned him onto his tummy and stroked him from head to toe while she again sang and rocked him. Soon Piers found that being in close contact with his mother's body was far preferable to being in the crib. He began to enjoy being cuddled, but he especially loved it when his parents swung him into the air and gently rough-housed with him. At these times he would gurgle and laugh. A beautiful relationship developed. Time proved Piers to be very intelligent. It is interesting to note that even when Piers was much older he still seldom displayed facial expressions.

Talk to the child, but do not overwhelm him. It is important to talk to the visually impaired infant and young child, but care should be taken not to overwhelm the child with too many words too quickly. Some people feel that it is helpful to talk to small children in shortened sentences of one or two words. While this may seem simpler for the child to understand, it is important for visually impaired children to hear normal language in complete but simple sentences with emphasis on key words. The visually impaired child is often more attentive to the words heard in the rhythm of a sentence than to the sound of a single word. To understand the connotations and subtleties of language, repeated auditory reinforcement is necessary. Extra assistance may be needed. This can be provided by speaking more slowly and emphasizing the key words. It is also important to pause and observe the child to see whether or not he is understanding what he is hearing and, if necessary, to repeat what was said or to explain.

Recognize that vision connects words with action. For sighted children, language and the impact of language are repeatedly reinforced by vision. Language is therefore easier to learn. The child sees who is spoken to, the response, and the action taken. There is an immediate connection of information and words. For visually impaired children, this does not always happen.

The visually impaired child sitting on the floor while his mother bakes cookies may hear the door open, his brother John's voice saying, 'Can I have one?' and Mother replying, 'They're not ready yet.' John says, 'Please?' Mother says, 'Don't touch!' ... a pause, a scuffling sound, and then Mother's voice saying, 'Carry it carefully!' John says, 'It's heavy!'

The sighted child sitting on the floor in the kitchen while his mother bakes cookies has the opportunity to see and hear the door open, see his brother John carrying his gym bag come into the kitchen, and ask his mother, 'Can I have one?' Mother replies, 'They're not ready yet.' John smiles sweetly and says, 'Please?' John reaches out to pick up one of the cookies cooling on a wire tray. Mother says, 'Don't touch!' John pulls a face, does not take a cookie, grabs his gym bag, and drags it after him to the kitchen door. Mother says, 'Carry it carefully!' John picks up the bag, but complains, 'It's heavy!'

Slow down and give the child time to connect words to actions or other sentences. Complete sentences, provided they are connected and meaningful, are usually not a problem for visually impaired children. However, caregivers must make allowances for the additional time that will be required if the visually impaired child is to make the necessary connections between words, people, objects, activities, experiences, and other sentences. They should also be aware that sometimes it is their own interactions that prevent the child from connecting words to activities. The following situation can show how easily this can happen.

Hedy had no vision. One day when she was eighteen months old her aunt filmed her using her new video camera. Hedy was sitting on her mother's knee. 'Where is your nose, Hedy?' asked her mother. Hedy slowly touched her nose. 'That's right,' her mother said. 'Can you find your hair?' Before Hedy could respond she heard her father's voice. 'Show us your ears, Hedy. She showed me her ears this morning,' he said.

Hedy was still trying to decide whether she should touch her hair or her ears and on whose voice she should concentrate when her grandmother came over. 'She knows her body parts,' her grandmother said. 'Come on over to Grandma. I'm going to give you a big hug.' Hedy's grandmother lifted her off her mother's knee and went to the rocking-chair. She didn't give Hedy a hug. Instead she put Hedy on her knee, and jogged her up and down singing, 'Ride-a-cock-horse to Banbury Cross.'

At that moment Hedy's older brother came in. 'Hi, Hedy,' he said, and without pausing addressed the rest of his remarks to his grandmother. Without a word, Hedy was placed on the floor between the chesterfield and the coffee-table while her grandmother went off with her grandson to respond to his needs. Hedy reached out, exploring with her hands, and came in contact with an envelope on the table. Her face showed interest when she touched it and it made a crackling noise. Before she could explore it further her father's voice interrupted, 'Whatcha got there, Hedy? Come over and give your Daddy five big ones.' Just then Hedy's brother returned, switched on the TV, and the filming stopped. Later as the family watched the video film, Hedy's aunt noted with surprise that with the exception of the first request for Hedy to touch her nose, nothing was followed through.

Hedy had very little opportunity to make accurate connections. She was not given enough time to follow through the instructions, so the words she heard did not accurately match what she was experiencing. 'I'm going to give you a big hug' instead became 'Ride-a-cock-horse.' The words 'Ride-a-cock-horse' were not meaningful, although they could be considered to match the action. 'I'm going to give you a big hug' was left hanging. When Hedy was showing an interest in the sound the paper envelope made, the words 'Whatcha got there, Hedy?' were tied to 'Come over here and give your Daddy five big ones.' Words and actions were completely mismatched. If he had slowed down and observed Hedy, her father would have seen that her interest at that moment was in the sound of the crackling paper. He could then have directed his comments to reflect her interest, for example, 'Your fingers have found an envelope. If you touch it again it will make that nice crackling sound.'

Hedy was an intelligent child. However, her language development was very slow. Although she could say a few words, she was three-and-a-half years old before she used any meaningful expressive language, and it was a full year later before one could have even a simple conversation with her. Hedy at eighteen months was receiving confusing information, so it was taking her a long time to make connections, and she required special help to catch up. It also took a long time for Hedy's caregivers to recognize how they were contributing unintentionally to her difficulties. Confusion is very common and may help to explain why language development is seriously delayed for some visually impaired children. It should be noted that visually impaired children can frequently memorize very lengthy sentences. It is making the connections that slows down language development and jeopardizes meaningful communications.

Practise using specific speech. Another area that needs to be considered is learning to be specific when speaking. This does not always come naturally. During the early months when an infant's basic needs are to be fed and cuddled, families can help their child by starting to train themselves to speak specifically. Instead of using words such as 'here' or 'there,' they can practise naming the place, object, or person being referred to. At first such careful attention to detail will seem strange, but it becomes much easier with practice, especially if the family works at it together. Learning words and how to use them effectively will be much simpler for a visually impaired child if he does not need to start by trying to understand these visual terms. As the child matures and words become connected and meaningful, such terms as 'here' and 'there' will be understood and even used by the child. Teachers of visually impaired, developmentally delayed children would make it easier for their students if they too were to practise using specific speech in their classrooms.

Use words such as 'see' or 'look.' With so much emphasis on detail readers may wonder if they should use words such as 'see' or 'look,' as these terms seem to be especially visual. In fact, they are no more visual than many of our other words and can be used in speaking to a visually impaired child. Blind people do 'see,' but not with their eyes. We speak of blind children seeing with their fingers or feet. Blind children quite naturally and correctly will say, 'I saw Daddy out in the garden,' or some other similar remark, meaning they knew he was there, heard him, or spoke to him. The confusion arises when the word 'see,' for example, is thought of only in connection with the eyes. However, it can also mean to perceive with the mind, to ascertain or comprehend – for example, 'I see what you mean.'

Include visually impaired children in conversations, even when they are non-verbal. There is a tendency to assume a non-verbal child is un-interested or does not understand. This is primarily because of our own need for immediate feedback. When we do not receive feedback, we think the system has broken down and have difficulty interacting.

> While visiting a visually impaired child, Felicity met an extremely attractive young woman, the child's cousin. Assuming her to be much younger than she was, she asked the young woman her age. The young woman, who was severely handicapped, was very pleased to be spoken to. With great effort she managed the word 'twenty' and then lifted a finger for 'one.' Obviously pleased to have been addressed, she went over to join in the conversation. Slowly and deliberately she struggled twice to make comments. She was reassured that her comments were welcome and that she would have time to make them. What she said revealed her complete understanding of and interest in the conversation. On two other occasions she attempted conversation, but was not under-stood. She was given time to try again, but remained silent. Through eye contact she indicated it was too difficult and wished to let it pass. Her joy and satisfaction at being included was evident. When Felicity left, the young woman smiled her pleasure at their meeting and then pointed to her head and said that she was pleased not to have been thought of as stupid. This young woman was sighted. Would there have been a difference if she had been visually impaired and less attractive?

It is important to start early to include the visually impaired child in all family conversations. This is particularly true if you are talking about the child. Including him acknowledges and confirms his iden-tity. Vision constantly reinforces the sighted child's identity as an autonomous being. Talking about the child's experiences in his pres-ence – providing he is included – helps him to rethink those experi-ences, even though they may not have been pleasant, and perhaps fill in missing parts. Through vision, sighted children have many oppor-tunities to be reminded of or to compare experiences. Remarks in the conversation such as, 'You remember that, Tanya, don't you?' or 'That's what happened, wasn't it, Gordon?' help the child to feel included. Another important reason for discussing the child's experiences in his presence is that it offers him an opportunity to practise listening and concentrating. This is so much easier for the sighted child who can see the person speaking and the visual communication, gestures, expressions, etc. For the sighted child there is greater motivation to keep listening. For the visually impaired child, his own experiences provide the interest and motivation. Regardless of the degree of the child's disability, treat the child as if he were hearing and feeling. When the child is confident, feels he belongs, and is considered part of the family or group, it opens the door to participation at whatever level. It encourages the child to join in the family or group interactions.

Learn the art of tuning in and turn-taking. Turn-taking is an art and for many requires practice. To be a successful communicator requires self-discipline and concentration. To be quiet and listen before jumping in with what you would like to say is not always easy. Tuning in and turn-taking also have the additional advantage of helping to prevent the learned helplessness or conditioned helplessness of the child who always waits to be prompted and who seldom initiates a conversation or an action independently.

Many families have never learned to listen to each other. Teenagers say, 'My parents never listen to me,' and parents say the same of them! It is actually a breakdown in the turn-taking system. Hurt feelings and misunderstandings are common. It has been suggested that TV, videos, and electronic equipment all contribute towards the lack of communication in families. This may be true and certainly for the visually impaired preschooler, music is often used so much that opportunities to practise communication are lost. When tuning in and turn-taking are understood and practised, many communication problems dissolve. In Chapter 10 we have explained in detail this important technique, which should begin when the child is still an infant.

Minimize nonsense or meaningless rhymes. Adapt or make up rhymes to match experience. Some visually impaired children learn to speak, but cannot converse. They may even have prolific language, but it is usually rote-learned, for example, counting, rhymes, jingles, songs, and meaningless dialogue. Sometimes it is in long sentences, or even whole paragraphs, but only a small portion of what is said is actually understood. The pleasure the child derives from repeating words is mainly due to the rhythm the words make when strung together or the reaction received from others.

Playing with words and sounds needs to be encouraged, as this is how small children begin learning to talk. Through making sounds, saying words, and reciting rhymes, they gain confidence. As words are connected to people, objects, and actions, language develops appropriately. Special care must be taken with visually impaired children to ensure that words are related to the child's experiences, so that they can be understood and used in a meaningful way. Until a visually impaired child can converse meaningfully, avoid using too many nonsense rhymes. Words can still be in the form of singing. Any made-up or adapted rhymes can be used, provided they accurately match the child's actions. Without this precaution the child can become like a language student or a tourist who takes pride in being able to count or recite verses or phrases in the new language, but has not learned how to turn this skill into meaningful conversation. Do not be fooled. Recitation is not communication. For some visually impaired children recitation may be the only success they have had using words to attract attention. For these children real communication has still to be learned.

Whenever possible use a statement instead of a question and build on the child's responses or statements. Consider your predicament if you are a tourist in a foreign land. You need directions, but cannot speak the language. What would you do? Perhaps you would point to something that would give a clue to your meaning, or you might mime, using gestures, facial expressions, and some words. Now let's assume you can see very little. Pointing might be difficult for you, but you can still mime, so you do. You now have another problem. You cannot see the passerby clearly so you are not sure how much, if any part, of your mime has been understood. What will you do? You can give up in frustration. You can repeat the whole procedure and hope it is being understood. You can shout. You can stop and listen to what the passerby is saying and see if the words sound like something you understand. If you think you've found some mutually understood word, you will probably repeat it, hoping that the passerby will get at least some of your meaning and be able to help you.

Can you see some similarity to the visually impaired child learning to speak? If he does not have the vocabulary, how is he going to answer the question? And that's assuming he understands the question. If he only hears questions, how is he going to build a vocabulary? We saw earlier how difficult it was for Hedy to build a meaningful vocabulary and we have also stated that it is possible to have an enormous but virtually useless vocabulary.

Making statements helps the visually impaired child to hear words (receptive language) and then as their meaning becomes clear to use words (expressive language). It is very common to start a conversation with a question. For young children questions often become the main focus of a conversation, yet questions can make communication much more difficult. If the child is non-verbal, knows a limited amount of the language, or is just non-communicative, questions are a foolproof way of blocking conversation. Here is an example:

Q. 'What did you do in school today?'
(No reply)
(You notice traces of paint on the child's hand and shirt.)
Q. 'Did you finger-paint at school?'
(No reply. The child rocks, twists, or just stands.)

As you can see, this conversation is a little boring! Instead you could try something like this:

Q. 'George, I think you must have had fun in school today. I'll see if I can guess what you were doing. I think you were finger-painting, right?' (Pause a moment and observe. Have you sparked his interest? There may be a slight smile on his face, or he may be standing very still listening in anticipation, or there may be no visible change.)
Q. 'I have found a little green paint, right here. It's still on your thumbnail, and a little red paint right here on your shirt.' (Give him a little tickle. Aim for a smile or a laugh.)
Q. 'I hope you had a lot of fun in school. I expect you listened to all your friends talking and running around. You had a snack and you probably had some juice to drink. I think you have been a busy, busy boy today.'

You may have spoken for one or two minutes, but in all probability your remarks have been relevant, you have been giving him words that both build on and confirm his experiences. Stop now and wait for a few moments. George will need time to think about all you have been saying. If he is able to respond, it may take him longer than it would a sighted child to decide what words he will use, and how he will say them. Wait quietly and observe carefully. George may not speak. Some blind children mouth words or whisper. Some non-verbal children, by a slight movement, may indicate they are thinking about what you have said. If you were talking about finger-painting it may be a slight twitching of the fingers. If it was a snack you referred to, it may be a movement of the mouth. Even though you may feel the movement to be coincidental, acknowledge it as if were deliberate, as indeed it may be. You could lightly touch the child's finger or mouth and say something like, 'That's right, you put juice in your mouth,' or 'You were painting with your fingers.' Perhaps your child's movement was coincidental, but connecting the child's movement to your words will still be helpful.

If he has not responded or is unable to respond, you could now make some connections between home and school. You might make the connection by suggesting the snack was a while ago and he could sit in the kitchen while you prepared supper. This offers you many opportunities to build information by talking about tastes and smells, and help and encourage him to find the cutlery, etc.

After you paused following the statement, 'I think you were finger-painting, right?' the child may have given a very limited verbal response, perhaps just two words, 'Finger-painting.' Now you build onto his words, which he has picked up from what you just said. You might say, 'So I guessed correctly, you were finger-painting. You put your fingers in the paint and then rubbed them on the paper. I expect your teacher put your paper to dry so that you can bring it home tomorrow. I'm looking forward to seeing your painting.' If the child can see colours, you might add, 'I think your picture will have red and green paint on it – just like on your thumb and shirt.'

Some totally blind children enjoy finger-painting for the social aspects and the feel of the paint. Others hate it. They don't like to have their fingers messy. If the child you are conversing with hates to have his fingers messy, then it would be wise to pick up on that point as you build information. You might say, 'I know finger-painting is hard for you because you don't like putting your fingers in the paint. I'm glad you tried.' Try always to empathize with your child – pick up on what you believe he really wants to say. How frustrating to have someone state an activity was fun when you thought it was horrible!

Aim to make your conversation sound interesting. Without the visual aids – eye contact, facial expression, gesture, stance, etc. – tone of voice and emphasizing appropriate words are very important to the visually impaired child. They add interest and clarify the meaning of what is being said. Exaggerated talk is not necessary. It would sound unnatural and forced, so use just enough to make your conversation come alive. Some people do this quite naturally. For those who tend to talk in a monotone or with only the slightest variation in their voice, it will take practice.

Do not expect or try to encourage language if the visually impaired child is bored or unhappy. The motivation to speak even 'yes' and 'no' must be strong. When a child is uninterested or thinks there is no purpose in speaking, trying to encourage language is seldom effective. Meaningful language develops most quickly if there is fun and laughter. Blind, multihandicapped children are frequently non-responsive because they are bored. Response is often more readily achieved with physical contact, perhaps gentle rough-housing or something else they enjoy.

Do not always anticipate your child's need. In the analogy of considering yourself as the tourist who couldn't speak the language, would you have made all the effort to mime and gesture to the passerby just for the sake of making conversation? Unless you were an avid language student or incredibly lonely it is very unlikely! Your need to communicate was the reason you made the effort. Many visually impaired children do not make an effort to communicate because their needs are always anticipated.

Victor had been playing outside in the sunshine. He came into the kitchen and his mother noticed how hot he was. She said, 'You must be thirsty. I'll get you a drink,' rather than giving him the opportunity or encouraging him to ask for himself.

Prepare the visually impaired child for social conversation. A mature, verbally competent, visually impaired child must have opportunities to practise conversation. To be able to converse meaningfully requires knowledge, and frequently some preparation is necessary.

Visually impaired Mercy lives in an apartment in a northern city. Her cousin, Norman, about her own age, is coming to visit. Norman lives in a warm climate, in a large home close to the ocean. Mercy has never been to the ocean and only very occasionally has the opportunity to swim in a pool. It is almost inevitable that Mercy's cousin will talk about his activities and his home.

A sighted child in the same situation would probably have had many opportunities to find out about oceans, hot climates, and big homes. Much of this information would have been incidentally learned through picture books, television, getting a suntan, and seeing a tan on others.

While it is not essential that Mercy understand all about Norman's environment, it will be helpful if she's given some topics to talk about with her cousin. She could be helped to think about big homes (more than one floor, like a neighbour's house), oceans and hot climates (always summer), the type of clothing Norman might wear to school (sandals, shorts, and a T-shirt), perhaps their mutual enjoyment of ice-cream. It could be suggested that she remember to ask Norman what his favourite ice-cream is. You could build on school experiences, suggesting that Mercy could ask Norman about his favourite subjects and help her define her thoughts on her own favourites to tell Norman. The information you build will be determined by the child's maturity level and previous experiences.

It is not necessary to spend time puzzling over how to explain visual concepts such as oceans, which would be beyond the young child's comprehension and not important. Mercy could be told that Norman lives where it is hot and sometimes humid, something like how it feels in the bathroom after Daddy has had a long, hot shower! The ocean could be made interesting by an explanation and an experience of its salty taste. Mercy could also learn that 'You can walk into the water, not climb in like you do your bath and the pool.' She could be told that 'You can keep on walking and feel the water getting higher and higher up your body until it's way over your head and if you could breathe under water you could keep on walking and meet all the fishes!'

Unless she was a very good swimmer, you could explain to Mercy the importance of keeping close to the shore where the water is shallow. She could be encouraged to find out if Norman can swim. Tapes or records of sounds can often be obtained from a library and ocean waves can be explained by sliding up and down in the bath so she feels the movement of the water.

Mercy also needs to be helped to think about experiences in her world that would be unusual and possibly not experienced by Norman. Ice skating; cold noses, ears, and fingers; the heavy clothes necessary in the winter; perhaps tobogganing or a mounted policeman. Mercy could be encouraged to think about the activities she, enjoys and what she might like to do with Norman when he arrives. (She may need some creative help in this.) She could be encouraged to make a little gift for Norman, such as a card of welcome, with a message in braille, if she uses braille. She could make cookies and fill a box to give to Norman.

All of this is part of developing communication. It takes time, but it is time well spent. Added information is always helpful. This type of preparation may help to make it easier for both children to converse in a meaningful way. It may also help to break the ice. It is quite possible that Norman, who is sighted, will not know how to relate to Mercy.

All your preparation notwithstanding, remember that children are individuals – Norman and Mercy may not hit it off. This would not necessarily be a reflection on Mercy's blindness or on Norman's insensitivity. It is very important not to try to force children to interact. What is necessary is that the stage be set, and the children be allowed to do the interacting in their own way. Adults should intervene only when absolutely necessary. Natural interaction between visually impaired children and the sighted is often blocked by overanxious adults wanting the children to act or react in what they perceive as appropriate ways. After making preparations, relax and allow the children to be themselves.

This point also refers to visually impaired children and sighted adults. Norman could just as easily have been Grandma coming to visit or even the next-door neighbour.

Gently bring to your child's attention actions that detract from easy communication with the sighted. There are actions required of the visually impaired child that are primarily responses to the sighted person's needs, and that have little purpose from a non-visual perspective. For example, turning to face the person being addressed, or who is addressing you, or being still when speaking. There are also actions that are important for sighted as well as visually impaired people, such as listening and waiting for your turn to talk and knowing when to stop. These are difficult skills for the visually impaired child – conversation is full of visual clues. Facial expression and body language are frequently clues not available to the visually impaired child. The visually impaired child has to recognize the pauses in conversation and needs to be very tuned in. Sighted people can see a speaker turn his head, perhaps indicating the statement is finished and looking for a response from a certain person – which may not be the visually impaired person.

Tuning in and turn-taking started at an early age will give a visually impaired child a good head start in the complexities of communication. Forcing certain behaviour in a dictatorial way will not help the visually impaired child understand why it is to his advantage to learn to act in ways that are appropriate as perceived by the sighted. Explanations related to the child's nonvisual understanding of the world will make him far more willing to practise and cooperate from his point of view, even on illogical things such as turning a face to the other person – turning an ear might seem more logical to him!

You could say something like, 'It's hard for sighted people when you jiggle up and down when you are talking because sighted people use their eyes, not their fingers, when they are listening to you. If you were looking at something with your fingers and it was jiggling up and down, you would find it hard concentrating and listening at the same time,' or 'You don't find it difficult to listen from wherever you are, but people who use their eyes like to see your face when they are talking to you. It helps them to concentrate and to pay more attention to you.' A child, especially a blind child, cannot fully understand. However, he will recognize that there is a reason and that it is just one of the differences between the sighted and the visually impaired.

It is important to be gentle when putting these points across. A highly intelligent, congenitally blind man, a university graduate, expressed his annoyance with a teacher who had insisted that he use body language that the sighted believed to be appropriate. 'It wasn't so much what I was being asked to do, but the way I was being told, as if I were an object instead of a person. It makes me angry when sighted people treat me as if I were a lesser human being because I do not "see" the way they do,' he said. This man's frustration was obvious and perhaps justified. The teacher was no doubt doing what the book said he should, but had probably not considered his student's feelings. Empathy is essential.

Be aware that clothing can be a form of communication. While this may not be so important in the preschool years, it is during this time that your child first begins to learn about clothes – his own and others', and special occasion clothes, etc. If he is inappropriately dressed, social interaction may be jeopardized, particularly in the teen years. A visually impaired child should have enough awareness of clothing trends before he reaches his teens to know what questions to ask regarding the clothing of his peers, and to make informed choices as to what he will wear.

Independence or dependency on self for a visually impaired child can be achieved when the child has mastered the difficult skill of communicating meaningfully. Language and experiences must be accurately matched and then each experience is padded with additional statements to increase vocabulary knowledge and interest. With increased knowledge and interest must come opportunities to practise conversation, which will eventually lead to meaningful communication.

Opportunities to Compare with Others

This section, which sounds so straightforward, in actual fact covers some very complex aspects. Knowing and understanding oneself. Knowing what others do and how they do it. Knowing what others think of you and why. Learning about social skills and sexuality. Did you know that sex education begins at infancy rather than at adolescence?

Knowing oneself starts with knowing about one's body. This is not as incidental for the blind infant as it is for the sighted infant. It is especially true if the infant is multihandicapped. Exploring his toes may be difficult, if not impossible. A visually impaired child may not be able to see his toes or those of his family, so it shouldn't be assumed that he knows they are there.

From the earliest days the infant needs to hear the names of the various parts of his body. Songs, such as 'Head and Shoulders, Knees and Toes,' are helpful, but not enough. He will need to know all the external parts of his body. Consider for a moment just the hand. Fingers, thumb, nails, cuticles, knuckles, palm, finger pads and tips, the heel of the hand. The fingers have names: little finger, ring finger, tall or middle finger, pointer finger, and thumb. Then there are the positions and movements of the hands. The fist, pointing, fingers drumming on the table, clicking fingers, and waving. He also needs to know which hand is right and which is left. Using the two hands together, we have other movements such as clapping and pat-a-cake. When playing pat-a-cake with your infant, it's a good idea to begin and finish with the word 'clap.' The child then learns that pat-a-cake and clapping are the same. For example, 'Let's clap our hands and sing pat-a-cake. That was fun. We were clapping our hands.'

The reader may rightly argue that no infants and few preschoolers have all that information about their hands or, for that matter, any other part of their body. They don't. However, we need to remember that 80 to 90 per cent of all learning is through vision. With this knowledge, doesn't it make sense to incorporate as much information as possible into early fun experiences?

Most of the knowledge a child gains about bodies is learned casually and confirmed constantly through vision – the mirror, seeing other people, hearing comments that are then visually confirmed: 'Ouch, the steam burned my wrists,' 'Oh, I hit my funny-bone,' 'I have a sliver under my nail,' or 'I've got a mosquito bite on my thigh,' etc.

Making moments meaningful is a useful point to remember. Those interacting with young, visually impaired children should train themselves to be very specific in how they communicate and then to use each moment to full advantage. At first such an effort may seem strange, difficult, and marred many times by forgetfulness. With perseverance, it will become second nature to say, 'Daddy's going to put his head right in the middle of your tummy,' instead of 'Daddy's going to get you,' or 'Grandma's going to give you a kiss on your cheek,' instead of 'Grandma's going to give you a kiss.' Mothers don't have problems in saying, 'I'm going to clean up our bottom and make you smell nice.' They could just as easily, as they wash their infant or child add, 'You've got poo around your scrotum and on your penis. [If a little girl, it will be vulva.] There, now you are all nice and clean and dry again.' Just as pat-a-cake and clap are learned together, so can penis, vulva, or whatever colloquial term is used, be learned together. Each time the child is bathed, he can hear the names for and learn to wash all his body parts over a period of time. Some may wonder if it is really necessary to be that specific. Think about it. When and how do sighted children gain knowledge about their bodies and private parts? By looking at body parts and seeing their own naked body in a mirror, seeing the bodies of family members and peers as they dressed, or looking at pictures and statues. This information can be learned incidentally and constantly confirmed long before a child reaches school and then onwards through life. *It is a normal and natural process* for the sighted child. It can be the same for the visually impaired child, but only if caregivers recognize the child's need for this information and teach it in a simple, easy, and natural way.

The body is a blind child's reference point. It is important that a child learn as early as possible the correct words for his and others' basic body parts. Initially use the word that is appropriate for your family, but as the child matures, he should also learn some of the alternative words.

- *Head and face:* Hair, forehead, eyebrow, eyelid, eyelashes, nose, nostril, ear, cheek, mouth, lips, teeth, tongue, chin
- *Neck:* Throat, Adam's apple
- *Shoulders to waist:* Shoulders, collar bone, chest, breast, nipples, armpits, underarm hair, back, biceps, upper arm, elbow, funnybone, lower arm, wrist, back of hand, palm, thumb, fingers (little/baby, ring, middle, pointer), nails, fingertips, knuckles
- *Waist to buttocks:* Waist, hip, tummy, navel, pubic hair, penis, scrotum, foreskin, vulva, vagina, buttocks crease, groin
- *Legs:* Thigh, knee, shin, calf, ankle.
- *Feet:* Top of foot, instep, sole, heel, toes, toenails
- *Body positions:* Lie on tummy, lie on back, lie on side, crawl, sit, stand with legs together, legs apart, crouch, sit, kneel, sit on floor cross-legged, sit on chair with one leg crossed over the other, head up, arms folded
- *Body actions:* Nod or shake head, blink eyes, stick out tongue, open and close mouth, bite, blow, swallow, lick, suck, shrug shoulders, straighten arms, bend elbow, stretch, make a fist, point finger, cross fingers, clap hands, wave, turn wrist, bend at the waist, turn to the right, turn to the left, turn around, bend knees, squat down, stand on toes, stand on one foot (right or left), walk on toes, walk on heels, sidestep, step up, step down, step forward, take a step, hop, skip, jump, roll, somersault, climb, fall down, swing (by hands or knees)

What about body shapes? Small, sighted children learn very early that body shapes are different – that mums, dad, brothers, and sisters all have characteristics that are uniquely their own, but are similar to others. By the time (and often before) they go to nursery school or kindergarten, sighted children know whether they are boys or girls, and this knowledge again is visually confirmed over and over as they hear the words and compare themselves with others.

In various places in this book we have emphasized the visually impaired child's need for physical contact. The more physical contact the preschooler has, the more easily he gains body awareness. The following are a few ways this can happen. He can listen to a weekend story while snuggled between Mum and Dad in their big bed. What more natural way to compare Mum's and Dad's bodies? Here it becomes unnecessary to discuss it, since the child can learn just from being close to two bodies. Daddy's hairy legs can be compared to Mum's smooth skin. Mum's breasts can be compared to Dad's flat chest, or the feeling of being small compared to Mum and Dad. Most children love rough-housing. Being swung in the air or wrestling with the various family members allows the child to feel his and others' bodies moving and to test this own strength and that of others. Taking showers or baths together, swimming with family and friends – these are all opportunities to experience the shapes and sizes of different bodies. An opportunity to hold an infant is always helpful. The visually impaired child can compare the infant's size with his own, with siblings, or with Mum and Dad. Helping bathe babies of both sexes is another way for a visually impaired child to learn differences in bodies. Body changes can be a difficult concept. Putting on or taking off weight is frequently spoken of, yet probably not understood by most blind children. Even growing taller may not be fully understood.

> A counsellor of preschool blind children visited a former client who was
> now in his teens. At the sound of her voice, he welcomed her. Finding
> he could put his hands on her shoulders, he remarked spontaneously
> and in surprise, 'Wow! You've shrunk!' It wasn't until a moment or so
> later that it dawned on him that it was he who had grown!

A congenitally blind university graduate remarked that something had come as quite a revelation to her recently when she was squeezed tightly into an elevator! She learned that 'people's bums are at different heights!' Sometimes the fact that people grow, that they are short or tall, is only abstract information. When this young woman consciously realized that people's buttocks are at different heights, she suddenly understood why one grandfather liked the low easy chair – 'his bum was lower down' – and why the other grandfather, who was taller, avoided it. There is always some way that information is linked!

Another easy, fun, and natural way for blind children to learn about bodies is to help with the laundry. As soon as your visually impaired toddler is able to help put clothes in or take them out of the washer or dryer, you can help him identify some of the simple pieces of laundry, such as his own and his father's socks, a towel, or face-cloth. He can be given a sock and told what it is – socks are also good for learning that bodies have odours – and he can drop the sock into the washer. When they come out of the washer he can feel them wet and when they are dry he can feel how soft they are and how clean they smell.

Later, games such as 'What is this?' (a sock) can be played. 'What part of your body does your sock cover?' (foot). 'What goes in here?' (heel). 'And this part?' (toes). 'This little towel is called a face-cloth. What do you do with it? What does this big towel dry? Your whole body.' When the articles are being used or worn, the information can be reinforced again. Somewhere between nursery school and early grade school, a child can begin to think about what parts of the body are covered by what clothes and in what order they are taken off or put on. Of course you can reinforce this information by naming the order or asking in what order the clothes are taken off or put on as the child is being undressed or dressed. 'I'm taking off your sweater, next comes your shirt, then comes your undershirt, and now guess what I found? Tracey's chest and Tracey's back.'

A further step in understanding bodies is to tell a child about different clothes or body parts above or below the waist, neck, knees, etc. These are all fun learning games that parents and child can play together. Remember, make moments meaningful, but never treat this process as a test. If the child hesitates, give him the answer. Gradually the visually impaired child will learn more and more about his body and the clothes that cover it and, most of all, he will have fun in the process!

If this information building is started early, it is a natural progression to begin comparing a child's clothing to that of other family members and the purposes for the different types of clothing. 'Mum wears a bra. Feel it. It's like two cup shapes to hold Mum's breasts comfortably.' When talking to a visually impaired little girl, you can say, 'When you grow up, your chest will fill out and you will have breasts that fit into a bra.' You can say to a little boy, 'Your chest stays flat, but it might grow hair, and with your shoulders, straight back, and firm chest, you will be strong like your Dad.' Bodies of both sexes can be discussed. Little girls can learn about underpants. They can be told that daddies and brothers have penises, and they need flies in their pants and underpants. A finger through the slit helps the blind child understand. Little boys and little girls can learn that mummies and sisters don't have penises, so they have panties without flies or slits. This is another simple and natural approach to comparing bodies.

We said earlier that sex education begins at infancy. It's easy to see that its foundation can be taught comfortably and without any undue embarrassment. If left until the child is a teenager, it will become embarrassing and the necessary touching unacceptable. As the visually impaired child reaches each appropriate stage, he has the basic information for later discussions about pubic hair, menstruation, pregnancy, erections, wet dreams, etc.

When talking about pregnancy, do not fill your visually impaired child's head with fantasy stories about where babies come from.

> One thirteen-year-old visually impaired lad was listening to a counsellor talking to his younger brother, who was also visually impaired. 'Did you know you weighed ten pounds when you were born? Feel, that's the weight of this big bag of sugar. No wonder your Mummy was tired. Imagine carrying this weight in your tummy.' 'Did Joe come out of Mummy's tummy?' the thirteen-year-old interrupted. 'Yes, and so did you,' he was told. 'Wow!' he said. 'I knew the stork didn't bring me, but I didn't know that. Wow!' he said again. 'Then how much did I weigh?'

Use all the opportune moments you have to make your visually impaired child's world meaningful. If you are pregnant, let your visually impaired child feel the baby move. It will be so much more meaningful and exciting when the baby is born. If there is a pregnant or nursing cat or a dog, let your visually impaired child feel her big abdomen and later feel the kittens or pups nursing.

If all this makes you feel uncomfortable, think it through. Your visually impaired child is going to need this information. Someone will have to teach him. Who better than his family? Where else, apart from the home, can he be taught as easily and as naturally? Do you want to take the chance that your child may ask someone else, or perhaps quite innocently make a remark that indicates his ignorance? That question or remark could be made to someone who is all too willing to show or demonstrate the facts of life. The result could be disastrous for your child. Are you prepared to take the chance that if your child is sexually fondled or raped at a later date, he may not be able to explain what happened because he does not have the understanding or the words? Sexual abuse has happened to sighted children and visually impaired children. For your child's protection, he must have information and the correct words to express it. As a parent or caregiver, do not let your feelings override your child's needs.

We write this trusting that our readers are healthy, well-adjusted adults. Incest or any sexually deviant behaviour towards an infant or a child of any age is a crime. No mentally healthy person would consider any sexual touching, fondling, or other such behaviour towards a child. Many children have been emotionally and physically scarred for life because they have been molested by family members, close family friends, or acquaintances. *Our remarks should in no way be taken as implying that sexually touching or fondling is permissible under the guise of teaching.*

Comparing yourself to others means understanding your feelings and recognizing the feelings of others. It means knowing what is acceptable behaviour and how different situations demand different behaviour. Preschool years are the years when the foundations for life are built. Not understanding people or their feelings can have disturbing consequences. Parents and teachers are disturbed when a young, visually impaired child appears to be sadistic. He delights in hearing someone crying or being scolded. He pulls hair, pinches, or bites with great pleasure. The adults' efforts to control this behaviour are all perceived by him as part of the fun, no worse than going down a snake instead of going up the ladder in the child's game of 'Snakes and Ladders.' This behaviour may stem from the child's not understanding that others have feelings and, like himself, have bodies that can be hurt. How a visually impaired child responds to pain may also depend on his understanding of people and people's feelings.

Seven-year-old Christopher raced down the stairs to greet guests. He veered too far to the right and crashed into the concrete pillar in the front hall. Christopher's eyes filled with tears. He turned pale and rubbed his head. He soon had a large egg-like swelling on his brow, but he did not cry. His mother remarked that he never did, regardless of how badly he was hurt.

Some blind children react normally to pain, while others like Christopher do not. There may be several reasons for this. Perhaps it is because they have not seen facial expressions or body language when they or others are hurt; they have not seen others cry, or the blood, the cut, or the bump. Blind children should be encouraged to respond to pain. Adults tend to measure the degree of pain by the child's response. If there is no response, an adult may not realize the seriousness of the hurt. The child can be shown how to respond appropriately to pain by making him aware of how and why others react the way they do. When visual comparisons are not possible, the child must have help to understand his feelings, the feelings of others, and how behaviour is affected by feelings.

One exhausted mother of a young visually impaired child told her friend, 'Avril has just reached the terrible twos stage. I'm worn out, but it's wonderful that she now understands that she can assert herself.' Avril was shouting 'No! No! No!' in the other room. 'I don't call this a tantrum,' her mother laughed. 'I call it character streaks. It makes it much easier to deal with.' After about five minutes, Avril came into the kitchen where her mother and friend were. She stood by her mother's chair. 'I'm glad you are here, Avril,' her mother said, but she didn't touch her. 'You are feeling very angry with me, aren't you? That's why you were shouting. You didn't want Mummy to turn off the TV.' 'TV?' Avril said softly. 'The TV is off and it's going to stay off until Grandma has had her rest,' Avril's mother said quietly but firmly. Avril made an angry noise, then lay on the floor and kicked at her mother's chair. Avril's mother ignored the kicking and continued her conversation with her friend. A moment later Avril got up and climbed on her mother's knee. Her mother hugged and rocked her and handed her a cookie.

'Avril,' her mother said, 'do you remember this morning when Daddy slammed the door and Mummy shouted? Even big people get angry sometimes. Then Daddy came back and gave Mummy a big hug. We were sorry we'd shouted and slammed the door. I think you are feeling sorry right now.' Avril's face was expressionless and she didn't say anything. It wasn't until bath time that night that Avril's mother knew she had been paying attention and had understood their earlier conversation. 'Daddy slammed the door, Mummy shouted,' Avril said. 'Yes,' her mother replied, 'Why?' 'Mummy and Daddy were angry.' 'Who was angry today, Avril?' her mother asked. 'Avril's not angry now,' Avril replied.

Avril's mother had made a moment meaningful. She turned a difficult situation into a learning experience. By recognizing her daughter's feelings, verbalizing them, and comparing them to an earlier family situation, she had given Avril a chance to understand herself and to recognize the clues that indicated how her parents had been feeling.

Visually impaired children must learn what acceptable behaviour is and be encouraged to use it. They should also be told when others are behaving unacceptably. Children learn and mature by comparing themselves, their actions, their feelings, and their thoughts with others. To do this they must know about all the normal, everyday types of acceptable and unacceptable interactions that go on around them. The child must have the information to make choices, including those concerning behaviour. Visually impaired children can very easily be forced into behaving like puppets or robots, following along doing just what they are told because they don't know the alternatives. When they know and understand that there are alternatives, both good and bad, they can also learn that there are times when it is acceptable behaviour to say no, to be angry, and to stand by one's convictions. Learning these lessons in childhood can result later in thinking adults.

There is another aspect that needs to be considered. A child needs truthful feedback about himself. Sighted children can visually compare themselves, their clothes, and their belongings with others and they will know when someone likes or dislikes what they have or what they are doing. A visually impaired child should not be given praise unless it is due. He does need encouragement, but praise for a poor effort is unfair to the child and can cause problems later on. No child does everything well. Through trial and error and comparison with others, he begins to have a realistic understanding of himself. It is a visually impaired child's right to be told the truth. With sensitive help and honest information, the child can become confident and develop a positive self-image. A visually impaired child must be taught social skills. He needs information to encourage his interest in others. Through comparisons he learns that everyone has strengths and weaknesses, abilities and disabilities. For a visually impaired child, independence or dependency on self will, to a great extent, be determined by the opportunities he has to compare himself with others (body, feelings, performance, etc.). Without the visual ability to make comparisons, he must be given accurate information and feedback.

Independence

The following incident illustrates many of the points discussed earlier. Joshua is moving towards self-dependence. He has been challenged and likes to challenge himself. He knows how to ask for information and how to give it in response to questions. He finds an opportunity to compare with a friend.

Aunt Mary was a friend of the family. Joshua is blind. From the time

Joshua was an infant until he started school, she looked after him for one day every week to give his mother a break. Aunt Mary and Joshua enjoyed their time together and now that Joshua is eight years old they still spend an occasional Saturday together. One Saturday after a long walk, Aunt Mary suggested that they have lunch at McDonald's. Joshua was pleased and said he had often been to McDonald's with his mother and could now manage by himself.

At McDonald's Aunt Mary watched Joshua order his hamburger, fries, and coke and pay for them. Then with verbal directions he carried his tray to the nearest table. Joshua had done very well and Aunt Mary complimented him. As he began to eat, Joshua said in a surprised voice, 'There is no ketchup on my fries.' 'Did you ask for ketchup?' asked his aunt. 'But there is always ketchup on fries at McDonald's.' 'No,' replied Aunt Mary, 'the customer has to put on his own ketchup. I bet your mum has always put it on for you.' 'Well, I didn't know!' said Joshua indignantly.

Aunt Mary showed Joshua the packet of ketchup on her tray. At first Joshua found it hard to believe that this little packet contained ketchup. Even though she showed Joshua, hand over hand, how to get the ketchup out, he still tried to turn the packet upside down and to shake it just the way he used the ketchup bottle at home.

Aunt Mary decided to help Joshua now and work on this again at a later date. She also talked with Joshua's mother and they both decided to begin to provide some practical experiences for Joshua that would help him understand that the same kind of food may be in different packages and how these packages open.

The next day Joshua's mother heard him talking to his friend on the way to Sunday School. 'Does McDonald's put ketchup on your fries?' asked Joshua. 'No, it comes in a little packet.' 'Does your mum put yours on?' asked Joshua. 'Sometimes, because I make a mess,' his friend replied. 'I think that's why Mum puts mine on and I bet I can learn to do it without making a mess.'

In your opinion, in what ways have expectations and attitudes helped or hindered Joshua's development?

THREE

The Forty Points

The forty points encapsulate the material in this book. Each point is illustrated with examples and anecdotes.

1. *Physical contact is necessary.* Most infants and visually impaired children enjoy and learn from being in contact with another person. There is security and reassurance in warm, non-restrictive physical contact. Toys or a playground are not always necessary. A body can often be an excellent substitute that helps the child understand movements and provide challenge and fun.

> Example A: On her arrival, the infant development worker was delighted to see Stella, a totally blind one-year-old, crawling independently. 'We are so excited,' her mother said. 'Let me tell you how her brother encouraged her to move forward instead of rocking in one spot. He crawled on top of her! John blew on her head. She felt his knees and hands moving and started to go forward with him. They had so much fun.' She laughed.

> Example B: Theresa's nursery school teacher found her visually impaired student worked much better when she sat beside her instead of across the table. She realized this allowed for physical contact that replaced the smiles and eye contact she gave her other students.

> Example C: Billy loved it when his family provided a human obstacle course. This was their favourite: his sister bent her knees to form a bridge and Billy crawled underneath. Brother Tom was ready on his

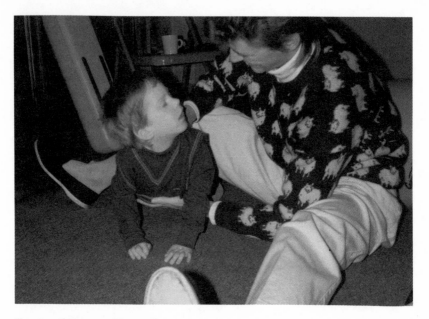

'I enjoy therapy with you!'

hands and knees. Billy climbed onto Tom's back and rode across to his father who was sitting on the floor waiting. Tom positioned himself behind his dad, and with minimal help from his mother, Billy stood up on Tom's back. From there he climbed onto his father's shoulder and somersaulted down into his lap. A rough-housing session followed.

2. *Before you touch a child, make sure he is aware of your presence.* The sighted child can see you coming. The visually impaired child may be concentrating on other sounds and may not identify those indicating your approach.

3. *Always identify yourself.* A visually impaired child may know you well by voice, touch, or special feature; however, he cannot build on this information if he has not connected this sensory information about you with your name. When a person is only a voice or a touch, it is difficult to call him or *appropriately* attract his attention. Identifying yourself to the visually impaired child is a courtesy. Without the constant visual reinforcement, the child may have an initial problem trying to 'place you.' Two people in conversation may use your name in reference to some specific situation. If you are only a voice and a

touch to the visually impaired child who is listening, the child cannot add to his knowledge about you.

4. *Use the child's name when addressing him.* To use the child's name is important as it reinforces his identity and autonomy.

5. *Address the child by his name prior to giving instructions.* This attracts the child's attention and helps him to differentiate your voice from the other sounds in his environment, thus enabling him to hear all of your instructions and not only the last few words.

6. *Encourage the child to use the names of others.* It is important to teach the visually impaired child to identify the person to whom he wishes to speak, and then to listen for a response before commenting or making a request. A sighted child can see who is present and what they are doing. Eye contact or body language indicates whether or not he has their attention. When a blind child makes a comment, it may not be answered because those around him may be busy and unaware that they are being spoken to. This seeming indifference to the child's effort to communicate may discourage him from making further attempts.

7. *When there are more than two persons present, or in group situations, use their names when addressing them individually.* This helps the child who cannot see to know who is being spoken to, when *he* is being spoken to, be aware of who is present, and identify the voice he hears. In large groups, when identification is not possible, such as in a theatre, church, or supermarket, the child needs to be told, 'There are many people here; we do not know their names.'

8. *Be aware that all language has visual connotations and may be a problem for the non-visual child.* A visually impaired child must relate to visual language that may not match his sensory experiences. For example, for a sighted child a description of a soft, fluffy toy with a cute expression offers a visually appealing picture. However, for the visually impaired child the words 'soft' and 'fluffy' may not have the same appeal; in fact they may represent something that he has found to be tickly or irritating.

9. *Make directions clear and concise.* 'Put it on the table' is more appropriate than tapping the table and saying, 'Put it here.' To point and

say to a partially sighted child, 'Go over there to Johnny,' when Johnny may be no more than a coloured blob in a sea of other coloured blobs, is not very helpful. However, to point and say, 'Go over there to Johnny. He's standing by the bookcase,' is much clearer. The pointing leads the child in the right direction; the bookcase, being a permanent and familiar reference point, makes locating Johnny a simpler task. A simple statement such as, 'Step forward onto your right foot,' is easily understood by the sighted child. It has caused confusion for some visually impaired children who moved forward with the right foot, then placed the left foot on top of the right foot, exactly as described.

10. *Do not ooververbalize. Listen to yourself.* Constant verbal prompting can be distracting. Allow the child time to respond. Without visual clues the blind child may need extra time to think through your directions. Patience is needed as the waiting time may seem excessively long to the busy adult.

11. *Give careful attention to touch and tone of voice.* As the child cannot see your facial expressions or body language, your touch or tone of voice should convey a clear message. When used together they should be consistent. For example, an apologetic tone of voice expressing disapproval or giving a direct command is confusing to the child. A sighted child may recognize impatience or irritation on your face and is not surprised if your actions demonstrate this. You will need to verbalize your feelings for the visually impaired child if he too is to understand. It is possible to disguise one's facial expression and tone of voice. Be aware that feelings expressed by touch are less easily disguised.

12. *Prolonged periods of echolalia (parroting) are common to blind children.* A conversation with Ruthy usually went as follows:

> Teacher: 'Hello, Ruthy.'
> Ruthy: 'Hello, Ruthy.'
> Teacher: 'How are you today?'
> Ruthy: 'How are you today?'
> Teacher: 'Shall we go for a walk?'
> Ruthy: 'Shall we go for a walk?'

Until the child understands himself and others as being separate units capable of interacting independently with each other and the environment, echolalia will continue. The sighted child has opportunities to observe responses to questions and requests and make the appropriate connections. Until his parents began role-modelling, Johnny would ask for a drink by saying, 'Do you want a drink, Johnny?' One way to make the connections for the blind child may be modelling questions and answers as follows:

Mother to father: 'Dad, do you want a drink of juice?'
Father to mother: 'Yes, I'd like a drink of juice.'
Mother to child: 'Johnny, would you like a drink of juice?'
(Wait a few moments, then, if necessary, father prompts child to give appropriate response. Both receive juice.)

13. *Visually impaired children need opportunities to learn to ask appropriate questions.* Sighted children have more opportunities to ask questions. They see a cookie jar and are quite likely to ask for a cookie. Visually impaired children may not even be aware the cookie jar is there.

Adults tend to anticipate the needs of the visually impaired child, which denies him the experience of asking questions and hearing the answers. With limited ability to observe, the visually impaired child will have to ask more questions than the sighted child to gain information about people, activities, and the environment, but may be less motivated to do so.

Example A: Whenever Sonia's mother took her shopping, she sat quietly enjoying the ride in the cart. One day a friend's child joined them. Three-year-old Alice constantly asked questions and wanted something to eat. Sonia's mother realized that her daughter was quiet because she was unaware of her surroundings. On future shopping trips she began to tell Sonia about the store and allowed her to explore. Soon Sonia was asking, 'What's that? Can I feel? Where's the cold?' when she was referring to the freezer section.

Example B: Annette told her mother that she had screamed at nursery school and had to sit on the 'quiet chair.' 'Why did you scream?' her mother asked. 'Cos my teapot was gone and I didn't know what to do.' Mother thought for a moment and then said, 'Mrs Bowley was right – you shouldn't have screamed. Next time ask, "Where is my teapot?" If no one tells you, call Mrs Bowley's name loudly and when she answers, ask her to help. Let's practise. We'll pretend we are at nursery school and I'll be Mrs Bowley.'

14. *Always give accurate feedback.* It is necessary to give feedback to the visually impaired child, as he may be unable to evaluate his own performance or know what effect his appearance, words, or actions have on others.

> Example A: 'You rolled the ball well and it came all the way to me'; or 'A good try, but you didn't roll it quite fast enough. It only went as far as the big chair.'

> Example B: 'Bobby must like the way you have threaded your beads, one round one, one flat one. He is trying to do the same thing.'

> Example C: 'Johnny remembered what we had to do; two big blocks and two small blocks. You'd better check yours again.'

> Example D: 'Anna, Tammy smiled at your new dress. I think she likes it.' Or, encourage sighted Tammy to tell Anna she likes her dress.

15. *Facial expressions and body movements may be less obvious in the visually impaired child.* A visually impaired child's feelings are often not as easy to read as those of his sighted counterpart. The child's face may be less expressive and body language less obvious. A sighted baby responds with excited body movements and a smile when his mother approaches. The smile is especially rewarding for the mother. A visually impaired baby will also be aware of his mother's approach. Small movements of hands and feet may indicate his pleasurable anticipation of her touch, or he may remain quite still in order to listen to her movements.

When you are explaining something or telling a story, the visually impaired child may have an expressionless face and/or be turning away. This does not always indicate that he is inattentive. He may in fact be listening intently.

16. *It may be necessary to give verbal reassurance when not close physically.* The visually impaired child can't see your whereabouts or activity. Periodic comments will reassure the child of your presence and interest. This is particularly important if you are engaged in a quiet activity, such as sewing or reading.

17. *When naming an object for a young visually impaired child, it is neces-sary to differentiate between the representation and the real thing.* Until the child has an understanding of the real thing, or a foundational con-cept on which to build information, a simple precaution is to refer to representations with words such as 'pretend' or 'toy.' For example, a toy dog does not represent the hairy, bouncy, noisy, sometimes wet, aromatic, and unpredictable mound of energy – a real dog – that may knock you over.

> A three-year-old blind child was used to his mother offering him new tastes. One day at the table his mother asked, 'Tommy, would you like a pickle?' The child replied in the affirmative. When his mother gave him a pickle he was angry and left the table shouting 'Pickle, pickle!' His mother was totally confused by her son's unusual reaction. Two weeks later she understood. At the nursery school the teacher said, 'Why don't you go and get the pickle to show your Mummy?' The pickle was a ride-on plastic toy painted to look like a pickle!

18. *Verbal descriptions must be linked to meaningful experiences.* For a congenitally blind child to internalize words and develop meaningful language, he must hear the words repeatedly in connection with objects, actions, and experiences. If this happens consistently, the child will understand language and learn to use it effectively. For example, to tell a visually impaired child that his friend is going down the slide on his tummy has little meaning unless the child has first experienced the slide, and has been shown what 'going down on your tummy' means.

> Whenever Simon heard the kettle he would say, 'That's the kettle boil-ing.' At a later date his family was astonished to find out that Simon did not know what boiling meant, or even what a kettle was! Simon had never touched a kettle or experienced filling it with cold water and waiting for it to get hot.

19. *Ensure experiences are linked to form accurate concepts.* A visually impaired child must explore the parts before he can understand the whole. Experiences must be connected before the world around him can be understood. When teaching a skill to a visually impaired child, it is necessary to ensure it is not left in isolation. As sighted people we forget it is vision that makes the connections for us. A visually impaired infant needs to have his hand in and on the dish

many times before he can be expected to know where the food is coming from. As he matures he will gradually need much more information regarding food, such as location, preparation, shopping, gardening, and comparisons between cooked and raw food.

Over a period of time sighted children understand the laundry process. A young visually impaired child will need to experience many times what happens to his clothes when he takes them off before he understands. He can help his mother put them in the washer, transfer the wet clothes into the dryer, take out the dry clothes, help fold them, feel them before and after ironing, return them to the appropriate place (drawer or closet), and locate them when he needs to wear them. As the child matures he can go on shopping expeditions to buy clothing and learn how to take care of his clothes, including sewing on buttons, ironing, and taking some clothes to the dry cleaners.

Five-year-old Matthew was totally blind. At kindergarten he did not enjoy pegboard activities. He used his two hands well, locating the hole with one hand and placing the peg in with the other, but he needed a great deal of encouragement and did not enjoy the task. His teacher realized he did not have the visual reinforcement that colour and pattern provide for the sighted child.

One day while walking with a group of children in the play yard, a student remarked to the teacher, 'We're back where we started.' She responded, 'So we are. Let's do it again and show Matthew the fence that is all the way around the play yard. We'll start at the toy shed.' As they went around again, Matthew trailed the fence and the children told him what landmarks they were passing until they were back at the toy shed.

That afternoon the children were using pegboards again. Matthew's teacher said to him, 'Let's pretend the pegboard is the play yard.' She helped him place the pegs around the outside of the board, comparing it to the play yard fence. Her plan was to make the pegboard activity more meaningful for Matthew and to give him a better understanding of space enclosed by a boundary.

20. *Know the child's eye condition.* Vision is very complex. Knowing the child is visually impaired is not sufficient. It is necessary to know the child's eye condition and understand what part of the visual system is impaired. This knowledge will assist in determining the most appropriate way of presenting visual information to the child. Correct lighting, as determined by the eye condition, is also a factor

to be considered. Some children may need sunglasses when there is snow and sunshine. Other children may require bright light. Glare should always be avoided.

Example A: Annabelle was multihandicapped. She needed a special high-backed wing-chair to support her body and head. Knowing she was visually impaired, her teacher used brightly coloured and reflective objects when working with her. Later she learned from the visual consultant that Annabelle had vision in the right eye only, and this was in the upper right quadrant of her visual field. Her teacher now understood why her efforts to encourage Annabelle to use her vision had been ineffective. Objects normally placed on the tray in front of Annabelle would need to be brought higher and to the right. After much thought a way was found to support Annabelle's head without using the right wing piece of her chair. Annabelle became a much happier but also a more demanding young girl!

Example B: Fiona's teacher found it very disconcerting when her young student turned her head away when spoken to, and chose to sit sideways in the music circle. After a meeting with the child's parents and the visual consultant, she learned that Fiona had no central vision. When Fiona's head was turned, she was using her peripheral vision to look at her teacher.

Example C: Trevor was an active child. In kindergarten he was frequently in trouble with children and adults for bumping into objects and upsetting displays and games. His teacher thought of him as a clumsy child until she observed how often he missed his place when running around the circle in musical games such as 'Duck, Duck, Goose.' She arranged for the public health nurse to test his vision. The results indicated a peripheral loss and Trevor was referred to an ophthalmologist.

Example D: In February the teacher learned she was to have a new student the following week. Patsy was being transferred from a grade one class in another town. The teacher was told the child was highly myopic (i.e., extremely shortsighted) and needed to hold objects close to her eyes. In preparation, the teacher made special worksheets with clear, enlarged pictures and letters. Patsy had difficulty with these sheets and her teacher wondered if braille would be necessary.

When the vision consultant arrived, Patsy's teacher was surprised to find her new student could read small print. Using large print Patsy could see only parts of the letters. The consultant also recommended a special book-rest to avoid neck strain and poor posture.

21. *It is very important that visually impaired children learn to use their residual vision.* Vision is both a developmental and learned process. A sighted child does not have full visual efficiency at birth. As the infant matures and learns to use his vision, visual efficiency is increased. The same is true if the child is visually impaired. For the visually impaired child, however, greater concentration and energy is required to interpret what is being looked at. Visual input may be ignored in the same way as some sounds are ignored because they have no particular meaning for the child. Motivation and encouragement are required to assist the visually impaired child to make sense of the blurred or fragmented images he may see. This situation can be compared to a driver of a car on a foggy day. He is motivated to see in order to drive safely. He will work at identifying landmarks. The passenger in the same car will be less likely to do so. He will use his vision to note the things on the dashboard or at the edge of the road.

To arouse and encourage visual interest, provide bright coloured and light-reflecting objects, and simple pictures with good contrast and clear outlines. Place objects close enough for the child to touch. Mobiles can be lowered – the air movement they make may also add interest. Sound-making toys and objects alert the child and may also attract his visual attention.

Example A: Mother had noticed that Tara always moved to the floor air register. To increase her child's interest she tied balloons to that spot. When she stuck a few brightly coloured stickers on the balloon, she was excited to see Tara make deliberate attempts to catch the balloon instead of the random movements the child had made previously.

Example B: Mother thought baby Keith had no vision until one day, dressed to go to a party, she discovered Keith was attracted to her rhinestone beads. Excited by this, she later collected some of her jewellery and attached the items to the mobiles over his crib and change table. She was rewarded by Keith's increased interest in touching and playing with the now light-reflecting mobile.

Example C: To encourage Paul to search visually his nursery school teacher spread a variety of food items such as Smarties, jelly beans, and

Cheerios over the table. Sitting at the table Paul was encouraged to visually scan the table, find all the items, and drop them in a tin. She varied this game by sometimes asking him to point to or pick up specific items. Through observation she learned which colours and which areas on the table Paul often missed. Using this information she devised fun activities that gave Paul practice in searching effectively.

Example D: Susan, like her classmates, enjoyed riding a tricycle. To increase Susan's visual skills her teacher stuck bright yellow tape on the gym floor and encouraged Susan and her classmates to follow the tape. At strategic spots on the route the teacher placed a series of activities. This required the children to dismount and perform a variety of stunts such as dropping a ball or beanbag into a bucket. Each activity was fun for all the children but was designed specifically to encourage Susan to use her vision.

Example E: After she had removed several items from the shelf, her teacher found Robin was able to find toys more easily. The teacher realized that the outlines of the toys were now clearer and therefore easier for Robin to identify.

Exercises are available to help the visually impaired child increase his visual efficiency. Contact a specialist in the field who can recommend those that are appropriate. These exercises can be presented to the child through interesting games and activities.

22. *The body is the child's reference point.* It should be remembered that it is as much of a problem for the sighted person to understand the visually impaired child's world as it is for the visually impaired child to relate to a visual world. It is necessary to have a point of reference that both the sighted and visually impaired can relate to. The body provides this reference point. When used effectively and applied to learning situations, many common problems will disappear. Activities such as building a block tower can be made more meaningful when related to the body. The child can feel the tower getting higher if his or an adult's elbow is placed on the table and the blocks are built up against the arm until they reach the tip of the fingers. Bridges can also be built over the child's own or another person's leg, body, etc.

Location, size, and distances can be more meaningfully compared when related to a body part. 'The toy is on the floor beside your knee.'

'Before it burned down, your birthday candle was as long as your finger.' 'The garbage can is in front of you.' Directions can be explained more accurately when using the body as a reference: 'Stand with your back against the bookshelf. Now walk forward to the table.' 'Back' is the key word that will put the child in the correct position to walk to the table now and in the future.

Abstract words can become clearer when related to the body. A young visually impaired child asked to hold the dog's leash. She was told to 'hold tight.' When the small dog moved away, the leash slid through her fingers. The adult replaced the leash in the child's hands and, squeezing the child's hands, said, 'Hold it tight like this.' When the dog pulled again, the leash was on the ground. The child did not understand the direction to 'hold tight.' The pressure from the adult's hand did not give a message that the child could understand. The leash was again put in the child's hands, but this time she was shown how to snugly curl her fingers and thumb around the handle of the leash and told, 'Keep your fingers and thumb together like this.' Now, when the dog pulled, the leash stayed in her hand. The adult then said, 'You are now holding the leash tightly.' Now the child understood the word 'tight' because the instructions were specific and related to body parts.

23. *Make the child aware of all areas of space surrounding him.* We frequently place objects in front of a child at hand level, but forget the spaces above, below, and all around. Spatial awareness needs to begin early.

An infant in a high chair usually has toys on his tray. To encourage him to explore other areas of space, it is necessary to draw his attention to them. Noise-makers could be hung close to his feet, at the side, slightly above him, and so on, to attract his attention and encourage him to reach out to sound. In the beginning he may need to be shown how to find the object. Move the child's hand to the object – not the object to the hand. To continue developing spatial concepts, a child can be encouraged to find a toy that is behind him, on a high shelf, or at the back of the cupboard.

24. *After interacting with a visually impaired child, advise him when you leave or momentarily turn to speak or comment to another person.* Many visually impaired people have been frustrated and embarrassed when they found that they were talking to themselves. When interacting with a visually impaired child, a quick comment made to another

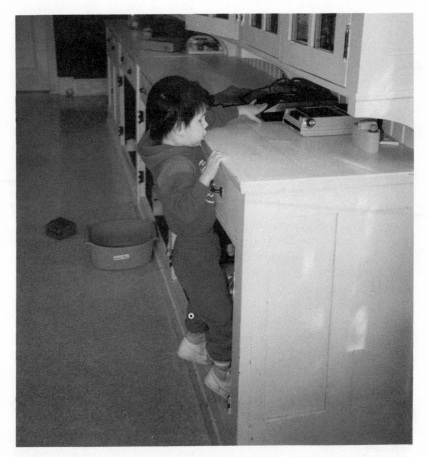

Stepping up and reaching out: blind children need to be encouraged to find things beyond their reach.

person whom the child does not see will be out of context for the child and therefore confusing.

25. *When you are walking with a visually impaired child and must leave him or momentarily move away, be sure he knows his location and is in contact with something.*

In a familiar self-serve restaurant June's mother moved to the end of the counter to pick up napkins without telling her daughter. Confused by the sound and being out of touch with her mother, June began to cry.

Her mother was surprised by June's reaction as she had moved only two feet away and had taken only a few seconds.

26. *Do not verbally or physically instruct a child to change direction when he is in mid-space.* When a child is going in the wrong direction, allow him to come in contact with an object. Wait to see if he corrects himself. If not, identify where he is and then redirect – e.g., 'You are at the climbing frame. The path is on your right.' Comments such as 'Turn around, you're going the wrong way,' are confusing when the child is in open space. Occasionally safety factors will necessitate directing the child to stop or wait. The child should be taught at an early age to respond to these commands.

27. *Right and left can be taught to many young totally blind children and those with very limited vision.* Blind children experience fewer reversal problems than the young sighted child. Learning right and left, along with body parts, can be helpful and natural to a blind child. A young sighted child, when facing and imitating his mother, will raise his left arm when she has her right arm up. Raising the correct arm is confusing to the sighted child because of the mirror-image effect. This is not a problem if the child is blind.

For sighted and visually impaired children, the word 'right' – meaning both a direction and 'correct' – may be confusing.

28. *Identify permanent reference points to facilitate orientation.* Permanent reference points will assist the child in orienting himself within his environment and help him to mentally map the area. It is recommended that all those who are actively involved with the child know and use the same familiar references when explaining location or giving directions. Permanent reference points could be a cloakroom, doorway, window, built-in bookshelf, carpet, linoleum, etc.

29. *Identify pleasant and unpleasant smells and tastes.* Smells, both pleasant and unpleasant, should be identified as they are important clues to the environment. For example, knowing the odours and tastes associated with food is important in order to identify whether they are fresh or going bad. If identified for the child, pleasant and unpleasant smells are clues to location: the smell of chlorine in the swimming pool or herbs in the vegetable garden.

Smells also indicate clean and dirty, such as babies, clothes, and fridges. Environmental information can also be learned by smell. For example, the smell of wet earth means that it rained last night.

30. *Note sounds in the environment and identify them for the child.* Sounds accurately identified for the visually impaired child help him understand his environment. He will depend on sounds to orientate himself; to identify and locate objects and activities; to judge distance, speed, and direction of movement; etc.

31. *Be aware that sounds can be confusing to the visually impaired child.* The sound of an air-conditioner turned on in a familiar store changes the environment for the visually impaired child. Some children may be fearful, while others may be confused by the noise, which may muffle the usual sounds that give orientation clues.

Sight helps a child determine the danger or safety of his immediate environment. At a glance the sighted child sees that there is no danger and may not even notice unusual sounds around him. These same sounds heard by a visually impaired child may cause fear or disorientation. For example, sighted children know there is no danger to them when they hear construction activity behind the wall of the play yard. This is not necessarily so for the visually impaired child, who may not understand where that activity is taking place and how it may affect him.

32. *Use TV, radio, and music selectively.* TV and radio voices usually use language that is unrelated to the child's experiences, which can cause confusion and discourage communication. However, watching TV or listening to the radio with an adult or older brother or sister to interpret can be a positive shared experience.

All young children may engage in repetitive language for a short time, including TV jingles. However, it is vision that attracts the sighted child to other activities and provides opportunities to observe the results of verbal communication. Visually impaired children will need to be directed to alternative activities. To be meaningful, language must be teamed with experiences.

Grandma was excited when her visually impaired grandchild began to use language during her visit. Six months later, on her next visit, she found a very vocal child but was concerned when she realized that his language was not understood by him or related to the questions and conversations taking place. She was told that her grandchild was quoting commercials and often repeated sentences from the TV programs. His mother had enjoyed the fact that her young son had language. Now she realized he needed meaningful language. She limited the use of TV and began to encourage words and songs that related to his daily activities.

Music is essential. It is enjoyed by all children and is educational and recreational. However, indiscriminate use of music can cause serious problems for the non-visual child. It may delay development in all areas by discouraging the visually impaired child from exploring the environment and seeking new experiences. The effect of this can be far-reaching, often resulting in poor fine- and gross-motor development, lack of purposeful mobility, limited social skills, and fragmented concept development.

A sighted infant or young child listens contentedly to music while using his hands to explore objects he sees within his reach, or he remains mentally active as he watches the activities nearby. By contrast, the visually impaired child in the same situation may find the music more interesting than the toys and people around him. The child may then begin to resent those who try to interact with him or feel insecure when the music is turned off.

If background music is on constantly, the visually impaired child, while still interacting with his environment, is missing clues that will help him to become tuned in and effective in coping with his surroundings. For example, the sound of a car in the driveway may indicate Daddy is home. Footsteps – even the vibrations on a carpet – can alert a child that a person is approaching or leaving. With the opportunity to do so, the child may learn whose footsteps they are and where they are coming from.

An older child who has become dependent on passive recreation will have little inclination to seek out people. Without practice he will have difficulty socializing with peers and making friends.

Visually impaired children will enjoy being actively involved in music. Use it to motivate, to teach, to relax an overexcited or unhappy child, and to encourage interaction and exploration. Music is the greatest tool! Here are some suggestions for using music creatively.

- Sing body-awareness songs, such as 'Head and Shoulders,' or adapt well-known rhymes or songs so they have appropriate words.
- Sing songs about what the child is doing, such as 'This is the way we climb the stairs, climb the stairs/put on our coat.'
- A distressed child in a unfamiliar situation may be seated in a quiet corner of a room. Music from a cassette player can be placed between the child and any disturbing sounds. Gradually reduce the volume of the music as the child gains confidence and becomes comfortable with the environment.

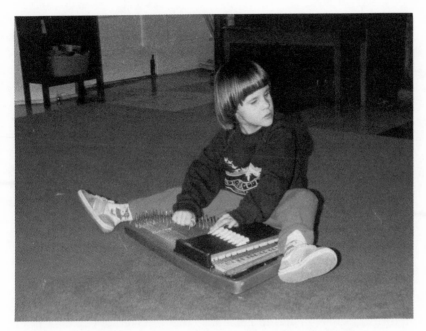

'Listening as I play.'

- Play musical games, such as finding an object while guided by the volume of voices (singing) or sounds (clapping). Loud indicates the child is close, soft indicates distance, or vice versa.
- Have the child imitate rhythms.
- Sing songs fast or slow.
- Sing rhyming words.
- Make simple musical instruments and sound-makers – comb-and-paper, shakers, clay flower pots suspended with heavy string from a broom handle resting on two chairs, which make interesting sounds when gently tapped with a wooden spoon (sizes of pots determine the tones).
- Find opportunities for hands-on exploration of musical instruments.
- Make tapes of voices and sounds in the environment.
- Add your own sounds in rhythm to prerecorded music.
- Teach specific body movements and dance steps to music.
- Before the music stops, find the hidden music box, clock, or timer.
- Children should learn to operate their own tape recorders and record-players.

• Tapes and the sides of records can be identified by tactual (plastic, felt, sandpaper, or wool, etc.) or braille markers. Also mark the switches or buttons to be pushed or turned on the machine.

33. *To facilitate independence, the visually impaired child will need more intervention and encouragement than his sighted counterpart.* A simple explanation of what is available may not be enough. Repeated and directed help to experience his environment may be necessary. Vision motivates a child to explore. When a child is visually impaired, he may not see the items that offer potential for fun, interest, and language. His ability to observe his peers is also limited.

34. *Be careful not to allow the child to function as an extension of yourself.* A young visually impaired child does not know that others do not have someone moving them around and physically prompting them. Allow time and encourage the child to operate independently. For example, after placing the cup on the table in front of the child, you may need to take his hand to the cup to locate it. However, always return the child's hand to his lap, so that to take the cup he repeats the movement independently. If you leave his hand on the cup, you found it – he didn't.

A blind child may require many experiences before he can follow a group direction. For example, a teacher announces, 'Time for snack.' All the children except the blind child move to the table. The blind child waits expectantly for an individual verbal or physical prompting. Delay your prompting. Allow the child time to hear the other children move to the table and their snack time comments. Try to avoid taking him to the table; calling him is preferable as it helps him gain confidence to move independently.

35. *Care must be taken to ensure that the visually impaired child is not left in a void-like situation.* A child must have opportunity to constructively and intellectually interact with his environment. This does not mean the child should never be allowed to relax and be still. However, to encourage interaction, objects should be close by so that when he chooses he can explore.

A small sighted child in a high chair can throw a toy to the floor, but he can still be mentally active and interested as he visually scans his immediate environment. With the toy gone, the visually impaired child may find no other external interest and turn to his body for amusement. If this happens frequently, repetitive mannerisms can develop.

36. *Learn to recognize when the visually impaired child is tuning out the world.* All children tune out from time to time and this is normal. If the child's world is frequently confusing or uninteresting, he may begin to tune out and find satisfaction in repetitive body movements. The visually impaired child may tune out more frequently than the sighted child because he does not see the many opportunities for spontaneous activities that are so readily available to his sighted peers – the box to jump off of, the obstacle-free hall to run along, Mother's shoes to try on, or the puddle to jump in. This lack of visual stimulus causes him to find substitute methods to meet his needs. Usually these are body oriented – rocking, bouncing, hand flailing, eye poking, masturbating, vocalizing, head banging, etc. Unless ways are found to prevent or curtail these activities, they very quickly become habits that are difficult to break and can persist even when the child is constructively occupied.

Although inappropriate, these start as coping behaviours for the visually impaired child. It is preferable not to reprimand the child, but instead to show how he can interact with his environment in a more appropriate manner. Give careful thought to your intervention. Unless the substitution is meaningful from the visually impaired child's perspective, he will continue with his undesirable coping behaviour.

Millie is a totally blind child in nursery school. When not interacting with her teacher, she would twirl in circles, jump up and down, clap, or flap her hands. The vision consultant gave Millie's teacher the following prepared list of questions, suggesting it might help both her teacher and family to understand Millie's behaviour:

- Is the child spending too long in the crib or in the same position?
- Does the child need more contact in the form of cuddling or physical activities with his family?
- Is the child getting enough physical exercise?
- Is the child spending too much time at one activity?
- Are there too many confusing sounds around the child?
- Is the child spending too much time in front of the TV, radio, or record-player?
- Has the child been introduced to a variety of activities?
- Does the child know what activities are available to him and where they are located?

- Does the child know that he can make choices and initiate new activities?
- Are the fine-motor activities meaningful to the child?
- How is the child being challenged?
- Is the child being encouraged to be independent?
- Does the child understand what is expected of him, or is he confused by visual language, mixed messages, etc.?
- Is the child being motivated to use his residual vision?

Millie's teacher and family checked the list and were surprised to find there were many areas that they had overlooked or assumed Millie understood. With their new awareness of Millie's needs, they were able to think through and remedy the situation. As Millie became more active, her twirling and clapping decreased. In a few months this behaviour was seldom seen except when Millie was very tired or stressed.

37. *Unconventional methods may be needed to motivate and interest a visually impaired child. There is no one right way. If it works, it is usually the right way.* Visually impaired children often lack challenge and excitement and become bored and frustrated with the toys or methods used by sighted people. To be successful, the motivation methods and play items used to interact with the child must reflect the child's unique non-visual, sensory understanding of his world. A favourite game for one young boy was when his father lined up in front of him various items from the kitchen cupboards. The child had to identify each item by smell alone before the bell on the kitchen timer went off. If he failed, a wet sponge was thrown at him! Not all would enjoy it, but for this child the game was challenging, educational, and very exciting. Water can be used in many ways to motivate visually impaired children.

A totally blind three-year-old child with spina bifida was tactile defensive – he withdrew his hands and cried when anything new was introduced to him. The problem was overcome successfully. The child loved fast movement. Unfamiliar household items were gathered together and placed close by. The child was seated on the lap of an adult, facing him. He was then swung up into the air and returned to the adult's lap. The child's hands were brought to one of the items, which was named. As the child protested he was immediately swung back into the air. The process was repeated many times. In the excitement of the game, the child forgot to be defensive. Soon it was possible to show him and talk about each item and then help him tactually explore it. The diverting tactics were no longer necessary.

Not all children would enjoy being swung in the air, but each child has something that gives him pleasure. It might be a simple hug or rough-housing, and will usually be body-oriented.

38. *Visually impaired children may need more support, but should meet the same behavioural expectations as their sighted peers.* Visually impaired children will need individual attention and some special consideration if they are to learn and function in a group. It is easy for the adult to forget that the visually impaired child also has a need to be liked and to feel part of the group. As with all children, he should be taught to have consideration for others, to share, to take turns, and to behave appropriately.

Example A: At story time Mandy was expected to sit quietly like all the other children. As she could not see or look around the room, she was given a toy to manipulate with her fingers. Her favourite was a pipe-cleaner or a small ball of play dough.

Example B: Totally blind twelve-year-old Brenda was visiting her aunt, whom she had not seen for a long time. At the table Brenda was pulling her bread and jam apart with her hands and stuffing it into her mouth. Her aunt gently corrected her, suggesting the acceptable way to eat bread and jam is by cutting it into small pieces before putting it into the mouth, or to pick it up and bite a small piece off. Brenda's response was, 'Someone would have told me before if it wasn't okay.'

Example C: Mark sat six inches from the screen to see the TV. This caused arguments as he blocked the rest of the family's view. After discussion with the family, Mark's father drew up a schedule that gave Mark and the rest of the family equal opportunity to see the screen.

39. *Virtually all visual concepts can be explained to congenitally blind children.* Sighted people are often sad and frustrated when they believe they cannot share with a blind child something they think of in visual terms, for example, clouds, colours, landscapes, planes, or bubbles.

Seeing visually is something the congenitally blind child has never done. The child has no comprehension of sight and therefore feels no loss. The child does not need to know what sighted people see, only what something being referred to is, and perhaps people's feelings regarding it. Obviously, an individual colour cannot be explained and there is no value in trying. Attempting to do so would only cause confusion. Although seldom necessary at the preschool level, the concept of colour can be explained. A cloud or plane is well within the understanding of many preschoolers. Rules of thumb to remember are: consider the child's level of development and understanding; build on familiar experiences; use non-visual terms; and eliminate unnecessary detail.

Three-year-old Theodora was quite satisfied to know that red was another word to describe her sweater. She liked it because people always told her she looked so pretty in red. When Theodora's understanding increases, she may need a more advanced explanation. The colour concept was explained to a teenager who asked about colour when learning how to shop independently for clothes. She was told that colour can be likened to the sounds you hear when you go to a concert. When the orchestra is tuning up the music is discordant. When the notes are played correctly together, the music is in harmony. Colour for the sighted is the same – it needs to be harmonized. There are some basic rules just as in music and, as in music, some people like one harmony better than another.

How might a cloud be explained? A congenitally blind child could be told that a cloud has many facets. If one is in a plane, the cloud causes the plane ride to be bumpy, so a cloud can be likened to wind or air movements. Clouds produce rain, so they can be compared to the steam from a kettle or hot bath, the spray from a fountain or a waterfall, or when one goes down into a valley and feels the cool, damp air in contrast to the sunshine. Clouds hide the sun and give shade. All, or any of these, can give some initial understanding of a cloud. 'Cotton batting,' 'white,' or 'fluffy,' have no resemblance to a cloud except in *visual imagery*, which the blind child cannot relate to.

You can describe a plane as something that goes high in the air, much farther than your arm will ever reach. It has an engine like Daddy's car or truck. You hear it and then the sound is gone because it goes so quickly. A plane does not have to stay on the ground. It can go high above your swing, the house, and the trees, and comes down to let people get on and off. Inside it has seats to sit on, like a bus. Wheels, wings, tail, etc., only confuse the issue at the preschool level, but can be explained when the child matures.

It is not necessary to exclude the child from all one's visual pleasures. If you enjoy a sunset or a mountain view, allow the child to share your pleasure or awe. 'It's so breathtaking,' you may explain as you hold the child or stroke his hair. The child can feel your pleasure and enjoy your companionship as you share the moment together. The child's memory of that moment might surprise you. It is quite possible he may have experienced sensations that could not be put into words, or sensations you were not aware of as you feasted your eyes on a visual experience – a pleasant breeze, pleasing soft sounds, a pleasant smell, or just being with you to share the moment.

40. *Be prepared for the reactions of others.* Not understanding the needs, sighted children may feel the visually impaired child is receiving preferential treatment. Encouraging discussion is helpful to all children, including the visually impaired child. Direct questions regarding the visually impaired child can be disconcerting or hurtful to the listening parent. A simple, matter-of-fact answer is often all that is needed to satisfy the curious youngster.

> Example A: On the first day of school several children came up to meet visually impaired Ronnie and his mother. One child asked, 'Are you his mother?' then added, 'Why are his eyes like that?' Before Ronnie's mother could reply, the teacher said, 'Remember I told you, Ronnie is blind. He can't see with his eyes; he uses his hands.' 'Oh,' said the sighted child. Then after a pause he added, 'Can I take the guinea pig out of his cage so Ronnie can see him too?'

> Example B: Three-year-old Tracey was totally blind. Aware of her need to be part of the family and also her inability to watch TV, Tracey's mother always held her on her lap while she and her two older children watched their favourite programs. One day her oldest daughter surprised her by saying, 'You love Tracey more than us, don't you?' 'Of course not,' her mother replied. 'Why would you think such a thing?' 'You always cuddle Tracey when we watch TV. You don't cuddle us.'

Small sighted children change activities frequently. They move quickly and may not think to tell the blind child what they are going to do. The blind child tends to stay with an activity for longer periods of time. Not having seen what attracted their attention, he cannot understand why his friends have moved away. It is unrealistic to think that the blind child will be able to participate fully in all social play without some adult support and intervention.

> When her mother reprimanded Carole for leaving Richard in the backyard, Carole burst into tears and said, 'Why do I have to stay and play with him? I hate having a blind brother.' Once she had recovered

from her daughter's reaction, Mrs Bell realized she was being unfair to Carole. She decided she must find another way to provide opportunities for her young son to play with other children. Some of her ideas were to have a popcorn party, a musical get-together, a dress-up party, water-play activities. For these activities to be successful, she realized that Richard needed preparation. The first of many organized activities was the wading pool afternoon. Mrs Bell bought a wading pool and in the next few weeks she taught Richard how to fill the pool with water and how to slide down the small built-in slide. Mrs Bell, Carole, and Richard played jumping and clapping games in the water to prepare Richard for splashes and for taking turns. Together Mrs Bell and Richard prepared cookies and juice. Richard practised offering them to Carole and Mr Bell so he would know how to offer refreshments to his friend after water play.

Mrs Bell and Richard decided to ask their neighbour, Kevin. Richard learned how to knock on the door and what words to say to invite Kevin.

The planning paid off and the afternoon was fun for all. Kevin asked his mother if he could have a pool party and invite Richard. Richard still had to play on his own, but gradually he was included in some of the activities of the neighbourhood children. It was a red-letter day the first time Mrs Bell answered the telephone and a small voice said, 'Is Richard there?'

Friends, relatives, and strangers react in different ways when they learn a child is blind. They don't intend to be rude or hurtful. In dealing with their own feelings, they will often be uncomfortable and at a loss for appropriate words. A comment intended to be supportive may sound thoughtless or hurtful. The effect on a parent will be different at different times, depending on how the parent is feeling. This is to be expected. It is natural that some days parents will not be ready to cope with people's questions and their lack of understanding. Some parents have found it helpful to have some short responses prepared for these occasions.

FOUR

Functional Vision and Creating Visual Interest

How We See

Light and the total visual system, which includes the eye, the optic nerve, and the occipital lobes of the brain, are necessary for us to see. Light rays strike an object in the visual field and these rays are reflected from the object to the eyes. The rays pass through the cornea (clear front window), the aqueous humour (watery liquid behind the cornea), the pupil (opening in the coloured iris), the lens, and the vitreous (transparent gel) to reach the retina. The cornea, aqueous humour, lens, and vitreous bend the light rays as they pass through and focus them on the retina (inner lining at the back of the eye). The retina converts these light rays into electrical impulses and transmits these impulses through the optic nerve to the brain. The image is received upside down because the lens has inverted it. The brain interprets it correctly and the individual sees the object the right way up. The eye collects information and the brain interprets it. For the optimum level of visual functioning, all parts of the visual system must be capable of operating.

Vision is both a developmental and a learning process for everyone. For example, a three-month-old baby does not perceive a plane in the sky as a six-year-old child does. He is not able to focus or track at that distance, nor does he understand the concept of a plane. In sighted children the developmental steps usually occur easily and naturally and learning takes place. As the child becomes visually aware, he begins to take an interest in his surroundings. As he matures, he is able to practise focusing, changing focus, tracking,

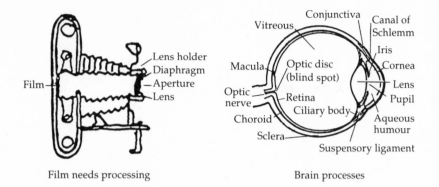

Film needs processing   Brain processes

The eye is in effect a natural camera. Shown here is a camera with its principal components and the corresponding parts of the eye.

scanning, searching, and eye-hand coordination. He begins to demonstrate visual memory and learns to recognize and understand what he sees. Seeing is not such a natural process for the visually impaired child. He may need to be encouraged to take a visual interest in his world. The visual developmental and learning process will be slower and there will be some problem areas, depending on the nature of the visual impairment.

You have a visual frame of reference and visual memory. Thus you can only simulate your child's way of seeing. It will not be exactly how your child sees, but the following will give you some idea of the complexities of visual impairment.

Light perception (awareness). You can simulate this by closing your eyes in a dark room or closet, then switching on the light. You will be aware of the light.

Light projection (localization). This is the ability to know where the source of light is. Depending on the degree of light projection, the child may not only be able to identify the source of light, but also be aware of how many bright lights there are on a lighting pole. A child with this type of vision may also be able to see shapes and shadows to varying degrees.

Tunnel vision. As the name suggests, this type of vision is like looking through a tunnel. How far the child sees through the tunnel will be determined by his distance vision. The size of the tunnel depends on the peripheral visual loss. This type of vision can be deceptive. In some situations it is quite possible for a child to see a small bead across a room and fall over a tricycle on the way to pick up the bead or be unable to look at pictures in a book.

There is an interesting exercise you can do that will help you understand this phenomenon. You will need two people. One person closes one eye and with the other eye looks through a peep-hole made with his fist. The second person stands approximately ten feet away and holds up his hand with fingers spread. Make the peep-hole just large enough to see all fingers of the hand. The second person moves his hand around and then uses both hands. The person looking through the peep-hole will experience how difficult it is to follow the moving hands. With the hand still and in line with the peep-hole, it is easy to pick out detail, such as how many fingers are up. This compares with seeing a bead on the floor. The second person now moves closer. The first person stays in the same position and does not change the size of his peep-hole. He now tries to determine how many fingers are held up in front of him. The closer the fingers, the more difficult it is. Only part of the whole is seen. Bigger is not necessarily better. Think also of the implications if the child does not have the ability to move his head freely.

Scotoma or blind spots. Imagine looking through areas scratched out of a frosted car window or stick spots of paper onto a pair of glasses.

Peripheral vision. If central vision is lost, try putting a large circle of paper in the centre of each lens of pair of glasses. You will find it extremely difficult to read.

High myopia or very short sight. Highly myopic children need to hold objects very close to their eyes and will see only parts of large objects – another case of bigger not being better.

Light sensitivity. Some visually impaired children cannot see at all in bright light, or have a great deal of difficulty adjusting from one lighting condition to another. Others are unable to see in dim light or experience night blindness.

Seeing with the brain. Many people understand in a somewhat abstract way what 'seeing with the brain' means. Felicity explains an experience that made it very clear to her.

'Without my bifocals, I cannot see very far, but can read quite easily. On this occasion I looked up from my reading and glanced at a tin about ten feet away from me that had been on the shelf in the same place for many years. To my surprise, I saw a very slightly lopsided but unmistakable face. I knew very well that the tin had a woodland scene on it, but I was now looking at a face. I put on my glasses and saw the woodland scene. There was a branch across the top of the picture. On the left, just below this, a large butterfly. A fraction lower, on the right, a bird about the same size. The shadow of the greenery was near the centre and below this, slightly off centre, a large bird. Underneath all of this were shrubs forming what had appeared a few moments ago as a jaw line. This was the face I saw so clearly!

'I removed my glasses and again I was looking at the lopsided cheerfully grinning face. I repeated this procedure four more times. Each time the woodland scene became a little more recognizable, but the face still predominated. The fifth time, I saw the woodland scene, hazy but clearly a woodland scene. The face had gone. I now saw a butterfly, birds, and greenery. I then had to consciously look for the face to see it again.'

This illustrates why in some eye conditions (e.g., cortical visual impairment) it is better to tell a child what he is looking at rather than asking him what he sees.

Visual Stimulation

Visual stimulation will not change an eye condition, but it can increase visual efficiency. Special visual activities are available to help the visually impaired child to increase his visual efficiency. Contact a specialist in the field who can recommend appropriate activities for your child. The following suggestions and activities are all related to daily routines or playtime with your infant or preschooler. Make them fun experiences for both of you.

Motivation is extremely important. There should be interesting things to look at in the child's environment that make the effort of looking worthwhile. Some babies and multihandicapped children like to look at new toys or objects, while others prefer familiar items. Each child's personality and interests are different. What is meaningful for one child may not be of interest to another. For example, it may be easier to encourage one toddler to search visually for a cookie you know he likes than to ask him to locate a block with a bell in it that he has shaken many times. The next child may prefer the block.

Visual functioning can vary from day to day and will depend on many factors: the lighting, whether the child is in a familiar or unfamiliar place, the person the child is with, the noise and activity level in the environment, whether the child is tired or well rested, upset or calm, healthy or not feeling well.

You will need to observe your young child and learn how he responds to visual stimuli. Your baby's response may be subtle – small hand movements, lying completely still, increase or lack of eye movement, or slight head movement. If you are the parent, you will know your child better than anyone. Through your observations and games you will be able to help others understand what conditions are necessary for his best visual functioning.

There are many good books that go into detail regarding anatomy, functioning and development of the visual system, common eye disorders, and glossary of terms. Five of these are listed in the bibliography at the end of this book. In this chapter we will concentrate on providing suggestions for vision stimulation that can be used in daily activities by parents and/or teachers.

Provide a Visually Interesting Environment

You want to encourage your child to look. Remember, the environment has to be interesting to him (not necessarily to you). Here are some ideas – don't use them all at once. Too many things at the same time can be confusing. In fact you may achieve the opposite of your goal. Your child may tune out or stop looking. Bring your child's attention to the objects you provide. Sometimes a sound or movement is necessary to get your child's visual attention.

Small babies see objects best when they are close to their eyes. Experiment and observe at what distance and in what position your child becomes aware of an object. This will change as your child's vision develops. In the beginning, place objects where you know he can see them. As he matures and as his visual skills increase, place objects in areas that involve slightly more difficulty and that challenge him to move his eyes and head to visually search.

The following are some items you can use: colourful toys, measuring-spoons, bowls, fabric, wool, tin-foil plates, pots and pans, spoons, bangles, necklace, Xmas-tree lights, tin lids, plastic scouring pads, nail or vegetable brush, crepe or cellophane paper, scarves, streamers, balls. If items are placed close enough for the baby to touch, make sure that they are safe.

Crib. Colourful crib sheets or bumpers can be used. It will be easier for your baby to see a colourful toy on a white sheet. Provide different shapes and colours. Keep one favourite toy or object in a permanent place, so its position becomes familiar. Change the other toys for novelty.

Babies like simple geometric designs. Black and white provide a good contrast. A bull's-eye design or a happy face drawn on a white paper plate with a black marker can be placed in the crib in the baby's line of vision or hung from a mobile.

Bright and colourful mobiles attract visual attention. Make sure the mobile is attractive from underneath. Adjust to the baby's visual distance. Some commercial mobiles that move slowly or play music cannot be adjusted to hang low enough to provide visual experiences for the baby. Attach colourful or light-reflecting objects to the mobile with string, so that they hang low enough to be seen and touched. Change objects frequently.

Make your own mobiles from a dowel or attach a broom handle or string across the crib. Hang colourful toys or light-reflecting objects fastened securely to the dowel, broom handle, or string. The frame of an old lampshade can also be used to hang objects. A similar idea is to use a small circular plastic clothes dryer available in many hardware or department stores, complete with pegs to clip on the string and the objects. A cradle gym will also provide visual stimulation and objects to reach for. Make sure it is close enough for the child to see or touch with his hands or feet.

Bedroom. Plain walls and furniture allow you to add pictures, toys, mirrors, brightly coloured curtains, etc., without making the room look too busy and confusing.

Change table. You could put a colourful sheet on the table and a mobile over the table, low enough for the infant to see and touch. Attach brightly coloured stickers, pictures, or objects to the wall at the side of the table. You could use a small bulletin board and change objects on it frequently. Keep some objects there permanently, so that the infant eventually begins to visually recognize where he is, but change others for novelty and interest. A lamp could also be placed by the table. Use a coloured bulb sometimes.

On the floor. Place toys on a plain blanket close to the child, or provide a colourful or textured blanket. Prop a shatter-proof mirror up against a wall or piece of furniture close to the child. Use the frame of a baby swing and hang objects from it, then place the frame over the baby. You can also attach objects to a broom handle or string placed between two chairs. You may want to lay your infant under the table or coffee-table. This makes a good playhouse. Stick tin foil, a suction-cup toy, or colourful paper on the underside of the table. You can also attach string to the underside of the table and hang toys and objects in similar fashion to a mobile. The child can either be on the floor or in an infant seat. Attach brightly coloured or tin-foil balloons to an air vent. Place the child close enough to see the balloons moving.

Infant seat. Attach items to the infant seat. Place the infant seat in a variety of places in your home (preferably in the room where you are working), or outdoors, making sure there is something interesting to look at close by.

Play-pen. Mobiles can be used. Attach colourful, light-reflecting objects to parts of the play-pen frame. Tie a string or ribbon across from one side to the other and attach interesting items. Later, when the child is pulling to stand, place the play-pen beside a wall and attach pictures, a mirror, objects, or colourful designs at eye-level.

Stroller or carriage. There are a variety of commercially available stroller toys to attach to a stroller or baby carriage. You can make your own using the ideas listed in this chapter. Tie a favourite toy on to the stroller so that you do not lose it. Attach balloons or a colourful windmill.

Bath-tub. Use a bright coloured face-cloth and towel, some colourful toys to float in the bath. Hang items from the shower head on a long piece of string, and from the handle over the soap-dish. This is a good area for using suction-cup toys.

High chair or table. Place a suction-cup toy on the high-chair tray while the child is waiting before or after his meal. You can use a colourful bib. Use a bright one-colour place-mat in contrast to the eating utensils, a brightly coloured or light-reflecting spoon, a brightly coloured cup or glass, and a plain dish because a pattern on a plate or dish can look like more food.

Car seat. There are some good car-seat trays available commercially. Attach toys or interesting objects to the front strap or bar of the car seat. Cover the passenger seat back that is in front of the baby with colourful or striped fabric. If you use a plain colour, attach objects to the fabric. Stick a suction-cup toy on the window.

Kitchen. Have a cupboard especially for your child and use it to store safe toys and articles, pots and pans, plastic dishes, dish mop, sponge, and a wooden spoon. Attach a colourful article to the door handle or paint the door a contrasting colour to the rest of kitchen. Alternatively, add colourful fabric or a picture.

Toy shelves. Using toy shelves instead of a toy-box encourages your child to search visually for a toy. Try to keep the shelves from becoming too cluttered. Keep only the current favourites on the shelves. Allow the child to help you change the toys from time to time. Sometimes the child should assist in putting toys back on the shelves at clean-up time. Shelves help him learn that objects stay in the place you leave them. He will also begin to remember on which self he puts his favourite toy.

Some Suggested Activities

At first your child may not seem to respond visually. Give him lots of time to focus. It may be necessary to repeat activities many times before your child notices the light or object you are showing him. Initially a noise or movement may be necessary to attract him before you are able to get his visual attention.

Observing your child's responses. The following activities may increase your child's visual efficiency as well as help you to observe how he sees. If your child is prone to seizures, first check with your doctor before using activities with light. In a darkened room sit with your child on your lap in front of a TV screen or a bright light. Do this on several occasions. When you feel your child is aware of the light, move your position slightly to see if he moves his head to look at the light. His response may also be to close his eyes or turn away. If you obtain the desired response, continue to move your location. If you have a swivel chair you can move slowly and observe if your child stays focused on the light. When you know your child is responding to light, reduce the size of the light over a period of time until he is responding to a pen-light.

Hold the child in a darkened room and switch on a light. Does he respond in any way? Do his pupils constrict? Turn the lights on and off. Does the child look towards light? Try this with sunlight, overhead light, lamp, or flashlight. Sometimes try covering your flashlight with coloured tissue-paper. Hold a large bright object between the child and the light source. Is he aware there is something there? Move his hand to touch the object.

Using a flashlight. In a darkened room shine the flashlight on parts of the child's body or your body, on the wall, floor, or a toy. Ask the child to touch the lighted spot. Increase the lighting level in the room and repeat these games. Flashlight tag is a favourite with older children. One child has the flashlight and has to shine the light on an agreed-upon body part of the second player. The second child can move and try to avoid the light. Set specific boundaries and amount of movement allowed (depending on age and skill level of players). You may need a referee. When the first child has shone the light on the appropriate spot, it is the second child's turn to use the flashlight.

Using a blanket over a table or a large cardboard box, make a toy house for you and your child to play in. Put one or two familiar objects in the 'house.' With the child, hold a flashlight and shine it on an object. Talk about what you see. When you know your child has seen the object, encourage him to pick it up while you keep the flashlight focused on it.

Attracting your child to faces and other body parts. Babies are attracted to faces. A baby will enjoy lots of close physical contact and face-to-face talking in many different positions, for example lying on his back or tummy or on his side, held in an upright position, or sitting.

Change your appearance sometimes. Wear colourful glasses or cover the frames with tin-foil, use an extra amount of make-up, wear a hat or colourful mask. Put lipstick on your nose or wear a clown's nose. Make funny faces. Stick your tongue in and out. Play with finger and hand puppets.

Show the baby his hands and feet. To increase visual interest, tie a bright ribbon around his wrist and put colourful socks on his feet. A small bell could also be sewn securely onto the ribbon or socks.

Looking and tracking. Babies and young children are more responsive to bright colours (red, yellow, orange), fluorescent colours, and good contrasts (black on white rather than yellow on white). Direct lighting should come from behind. Avoid glare.

Hold a colourful or light-reflecting object in front of the child. Give him lots of time to look. If he notices the object, move it slowly to one side to see if his eyes follow it. When he can do so, move the object slowly from side to side. Encourage him to follow or track the object. Notice if and where he loses visual contact. Give him many opportunities to practise. When your child can track horizontally, try up and down, diagonally, and then in a circle.

Most youngsters enjoy watching a spinning ball. A ball provides good tracking and eye-hand coordination practice. Roll the ball slowly from side to side in front of your child when he is lying on his tummy or sitting on the floor. Encourage him to reach for it. Then try rolling it forward and backward. You can also do this in his high chair or at the table. Start with a large ball and gradually work down to a tennis ball. You can use even smaller balls when your child is no longer putting everything in his mouth. Play ball together.

Have fun with toys that move at different speeds, e.g., cars, trucks, planes, mechanical or wind-up dogs, birds. Encourage your child to watch them, follow them, and pick them up. Encourage your child to watch the family pet move, drink, eat, etc.

Reaching and eye-hand coordination. Take these activities slowly, have fun, and give the child lots of time to look. Hold a colourful or light-reflecting object in front of your child and encourage him to reach for it. Hold the object still. If he has difficulty reaching, help him by moving his hand to the object, not the object to his hand. He has to learn through repeated experiences where the object is in relation to his hand. We do not want him to learn that if he stretches out his hand, the object will move into it.

Give your baby or child an opportunity to look at his bottle before he drinks. Later, encourage him to put his hands on it and then to reach out for it and hold it. Give your young child an opportunity to

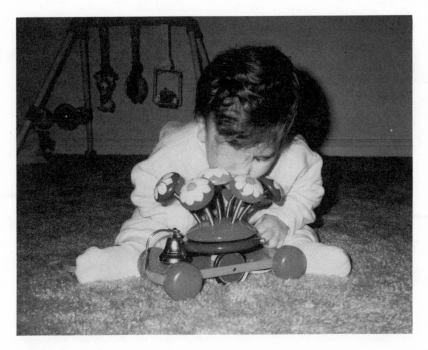

'What is this?'

look at everything as you hand it to him. Encourage him to look for a toy in your hand and also to give you a toy by placing it in your hand.

Drop blocks, balls, or favourite toys into a large bowl. Encourage the child to look for toys in the bowl, pick them up, and give them to the adult or another child. Try again later with smaller objects and smaller and differently shaped containers.

Puzzles are fun to do. Begin with very simple ones, using geometric shapes with handles. Use only one or two shapes on the board (a circle is the easiest). A good colour contrast between the form board and the space for the shape will assist the visually impaired child. Gradually add different shapes, smaller shapes, and shapes without handles. Later, if the child's vision permits, use simple picture puzzles.

Refining visual skills. Many commercially available toys can be used to refine visual skills – blocks, nesting cups, shape sorters, pegboards, crayons, and paint. There are also many household items that can be used.

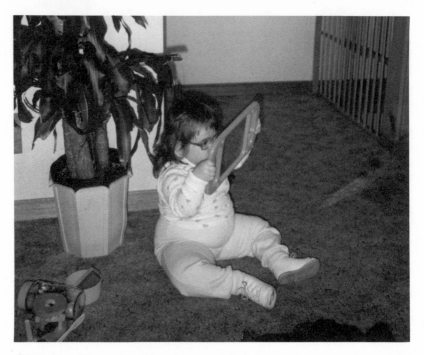

'I found it with my foot. Now I can see it!'

There are many opportunities for practising and refining visual skills outdoors – looking for steps; a change of texture underfoot; lines in the sidewalk; sunlight and shadows; shapes and contours to interpret; riding a tricycle or pushing a toy; following a white or yellow line in the playground; looking for garden gates, traffic-lights, stop signs, hedges, flowers; avoiding bumping into stationary and moving children; finding the toy shed.

Routine times. Opportunities for visual experiences and practice occur naturally at routine times. Here are a few examples.

- *Mealtimes*: using a black-and-white striped cover for your baby's bottle; encouraging the child to reach for bottle or spoon, to watch the spoon move from dish to mouth and back again; finding a cookie, sandwich, or raisin or a table, tray, or plate; feeding himself with a spoon, pouring a drink, finding his place at the table.
- *Bath time*: A good opportunity for lots of eye-to-eye contact; watch-

ing and reaching for floating toys; looking for the face-cloth, soap, or talc tin; encouraging your youngster to look at himself and at your reflection in the mirror; making funny faces, playing peek-a-boo using the face-cloth or towel; blowing bubbles.

- *Dressing and undressing*: Looking for buttons, zippers, pockets, labels, socks, etc.; looking for the top and bottom of a garment; looking in the mirror before clothes are on and when the child is dressed; taking clothes from a drawer or cupboard; taking shoes from or putting them back on the shelf; putting clothes into a laundry basket or cupboard.

Wherever you are, bring the child's visual attention to a variety of things. Talk about what he sees. For some children it helps them to understand what they see if someone labels and/or describes the object. Remember, things look different from different positions, in different lighting, and in different contexts. In some instances an object may be hard for a child to recognize because it is partially hidden or because it is being viewed from a different angle. Present familiar objects in a variety of ways – front view, back view, side view, lying on a surface, held in the air, or partially hidden. We all have difficulty with perception at times. Sometimes for us a picture may be hard to interpret until someone tells us what it is and then we recognize it.

FIVE

Practical Learning Experiences

It is essential that preschool blind children have knowledge based on a solid foundation of concrete experiences. A number of older blind children experience conceptual confusion because they are introduced to abstract ideas before they fully understand the concrete. In this chapter we focus on the concrete to emphasize its importance.

For the sighted preschooler, vision is the most effective source for gathering information. It is immediate and constantly reaffirming. Sound, touch, taste, and smell are all important aspects of the integration process. Without sight, touch, taste, smell, and sound are disconnected. Even though an impression is formed, it will not be understood until a connection has been made. Verbal information is not sufficient at the preschool level unless a concrete experience has preceded it. Here are some suggestions for creating practical learning opportunities for your preschooler.

Name body parts. As you bathe, change, cuddle, and kiss your baby, identify different body parts.

Name clothes. As you dress your infant, name the different articles of clothing.

Make tapes of your baby's sounds, first words, and songs. Play them back to encourage more of the same. Keep the tapes so that if he is not able to see photographs, your child will still have a memento of his baby days. You can also make a baby book. Attach objects to pages – for example, first bootees, hat, soother, spoon, favourite toy, a lock of hair after his first hair cut, an empty talcum powder tin for smell. Add names, dates, and places that can be read to the child later.

Keep a growth chart. For the growth chart you will need a long piece of cardboard or bristol board to hang on or attach to the lower part of a wall or door and a box of toothpicks.

As the child grows mark his length/height by sticking toothpicks onto the chart. While the child is an infant lay him on the chart and mark three months, six months, nine months, one year. Then mark his height on every subsequent birthday. For additional interest you could include the heights of other family members, using a different marker for each person, e.g., wool, string, or popsicle sticks. This tactual growth chart can be a fun learning experience for your visually impaired child.

To increase understanding of how his body grows, cut out handprints from fabric or corrugated cardboard, or use the mesh board (see instructions for making a mesh board in this chapter). Stick the handprints at the corresponding height marker. When he is older, he will be able to compare his own hand sizes and those of family members. The same thing can be done with feet. Later, depending on your child's medium for reading, add braille or large or small print, so that over the years he can read the chart himself.

Make tapes of action songs at a pace that is good for your child. There are many commercially made tapes that children will enjoy, but they are often too fast to make it possible for younger and multi-handicapped children to participate fully. On your own tapes, use your child's name in the songs.

Making a fragrant rattle. If you put some cloves in a child-proof pill container and pierce several holes in the lid, you have a rattle with an interesting smell.

Identifying and locating objects. Put bangles, boxes, face-cloth, and socks on various parts of the body, yours and the child's. Name the objects and where they are on the body. Encourage the child to take them off. Later put objects in pockets, cuffs, and sleeves and ask the child to find them.

Learning to sit. Before your infant sits independently, make sure you give him lots of different opportunities to sit with support – for example, on your lap, in the corner of the chesterfield, or on the floor surrounded by cushions. Place him in a sitting position on the floor and put your hands firmly on his hips to give support. Talk to him from slightly above to encourage him to lift his head. Show him how to use his arms for support. Make these pleasurable experiences so that he wants to be in a sitting position.

Using strong cardboard boxes, place the infant in a small box, one that he just fits into so that he can feel one end of the box with his back and one at his feet. This will prevent him from slipping. He can put one hand on each side of the box. Another way is to sit the child in the corner of a large cardboard box. This does not offer total support, but if the child begins to slip to one side, his body touches the box and he is reminded to shift his weight.

Learning to crawl. A blind child needs lots of encouragement to crawl. In preparation for crawling, a visually impaired infant needs to be comfortable lying on his tummy (in prone) – often not a favourite position. To associate pleasant events with lying on his tummy, here are some suggestions that may prove helpful. When you are lying down, lay your infant on your chest and talk softly to him. Roll your infant onto his tummy before you pick him up. Sometimes carry him with his tummy on your hands. When he is lying in prone on the floor encourage him to bring his arms forward; a small rolled towel under his chest will help. Once in a hands-and-knees position, he usually rocks back and forth, but seldom moves forward unless *the adult provides an incentive*. One method that is often successful is to place a towel around the child's trunk. One person stands with heels together and toes separated to form a 'V.' Place the child in the crawl position with his feet between the adult's feet (to push off from). This adult holds the ends of the towel to support the child in this position. A second person kneels down low close to the child and encourages him to push off. The person holding the towel gently moves the towel forward. It may be necessary to move the child's arms and legs to help him understand what is expected. Reward the effort with a hug or whatever he enjoys.

Another method is to use the stairs. Place an interesting item on the step above the child. Place the child with knees on one stair and hands on the second. Working from behind, encourage him to reach for the toy and show him how to move his legs to propel himself upwards. Remember to identify body movements as he moves up the stairs, e.g., 'you are moving your arm, now move your knee.' You can use the same words when encouraging him to crawl on the floor.

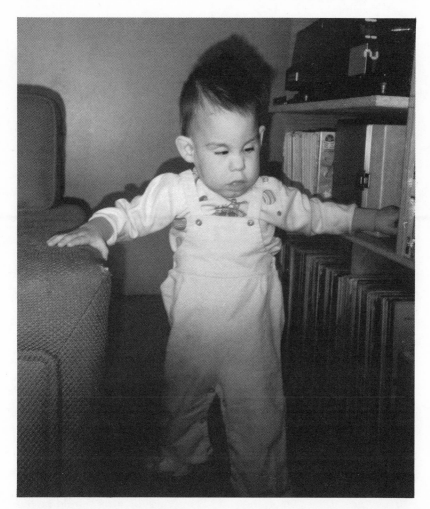

A safe place to practise standing – between two familiar and permanent objects.

Learning to walk. When your baby is learning to walk, place pieces of furniture a little apart so that he gains confidence in moving between them, for example, from chair to chesterfield to coffee-table. When he is moving confidently he is ready to walk within a wider scope beyond his arms' reach. Show him how to stretch to reach and touch the furniture he is walking towards. Encourage him to walk towards you and take that first sideways step into space. Practice will give him the confidence to walk on his own.

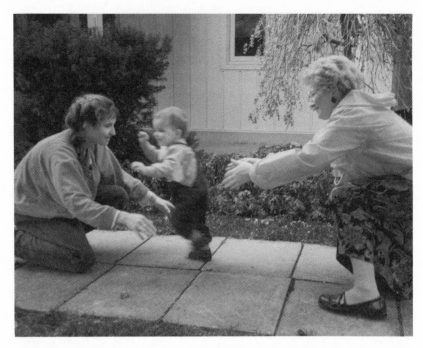

'My first step.'

The next step is to move forward. One way to teach the child to do this is for two people to kneel down facing each other, approximately a foot apart. The child practises walking between them. Encourage the child to reach to touch the person he is going towards before he moves. As he gains confidence, increase the distance, making it necessary to stretch to touch the person he is going towards. When it is too far to stretch, he moves towards the sound of the person's voice.

The voice of the person the child is moving towards should be the only voice he hears. Don't overdo the verbalization. Tempting though it may be, the adult should not move backwards once the child is moving, but remain in place until the child reaches him. As well as learning to walk, he is learning to understand distance. This can be a long process for a blind child.

Developing the use of hands. The blind infant may have to learn how to touch. Position the infant so that his hands come together as he lies on his side, or put him on his back with a rolled blanket or cushion under each shoulder so that his arms naturally come inwards. Blow on hands and other parts of the body. During routine and playtimes, make sure that the infant's hands at least momentarily touch his body, clothes, bottle, crib sheet, blanket, towel, tabletop, etc. Encourage the baby to find your hair, mouth, necklace, blouse, etc.

Children who refuse to hold or examine objects or use their hands to explore the environment are often termed tactile defensive and may have overly sensitive hands or skin. To overcome this problem, workers can try to help the child become accustomed to different sensations by gently rubbing the child's body parts with various textures. If the blind child has been tactile defensive from infancy, there is probably a neurological reason and these methods to desensitize the child may prove helpful. The child who will not touch what he is directed to, but touches and plays with things that are familiar and meaningful to him, such as a favourite toy, his own clothes, spoon, plates, Mum's face, or Dad's hand, should not be called tactile defensive but tactile selective.

When seen in a visually impaired child, often starting in the second or third year, a frequent cause is excessive hand-over-hand instruction with toys or objects that have little or no meaning to the child. It is best to avoid hand-over-hand direction. Use the wrist, elbow, or shoulder to gently move the child in the direction of the object and allow him to have control of his hands. Suggestions in the section on turn-taking will prevent and help to remedy this problem.

To encourage the use of grasping with the thumb and first finger, stick Velcro circles or attach clothes-pins to the child's clothes and have him remove them. You can also put pieces of sticky tape on various body parts. Also place rings on the child's fingers and toes, or bangles on his arms and legs. Encourage him to take them off. You can also make rings and bangles out of tin foil or pipe-cleaners. Encourage the use of both hands. Name the body parts or clothes the circle or tape is on. Put large paper-clips or clothes-pins around the rim of a yoghurt or margarine container. Have the child take them off and drop them into the container. Do not leave a child with these activities if he is still putting objects in his mouth.

Encourage the child to put objects into and take them out of containers. Think of how you can reinforce the concept of in and out through everyday routines. Containers can include cups, bowls, large and small boxes, large and small jars, bath, sink, laundry basket, bags, drawers, cupboards, car pockets, cookie jars, or shoes. Objects to use include balls, blocks, spoons, cups, toys, tissue-paper, feather duster, bells, juice, water, cookies, or candy. Hearing the splash as objects are dropped into a bucket of water is an incentive to release them. It is fun to reach into the water to take the objects out.

Noise-makers can be hidden, first under a cloth, then under or in a container. Several objects, including a noise-maker, can be placed in a container. Encourage the child to find the noise-maker. Later put lids on the containers. First use easy lift-off lids, and then try screw-top lids and jars with spring clips.

It is helpful to name the parts of the hand. If the child learns the parts of his hand, it will be easier for him to follow specific directions without needing the hand-over-hand method of instruction.

Compare bodies. Include sizes and characteristics of family members and friends – sizes of hands and feet, height, length and colour of hair, who wears glasses or has a beard or moustache.

Playing dress-up. Give the child a box of clothes to play with, his own and those of adults. Include an umbrella, some shopping bags, high-heel shoes, a briefcase, and jewellery. Encourage play in dressing up for shopping, parties, or Halloween; dressing up as a bus driver, a doctor, Santa Claus, etc.

Role-play. Your child will likely need a lot of help and encouragement at first. Use dress-up clothes and as many real objects as possible, and if the child is partially sighted, include puppets. Roles can include that of a doctor, nurse, or dentist, etc. Pretend situations can include going shopping, dining at a restaurant, going to the barber, etc. Emotions can also be a part of role-playing. Exaggerate facial expressions and body language, emphasize words that express feelings and show the child how to do the same. When the child has some understanding of role-play, take a more passive role and encourage the child to initiate the activity and be in control.

Water-play ideas. Show the child how to put the plug in and pull it out of the bath-tub or sink. Encourage him to hear and feel the water coming in and out. Show the child how to push a chair up to the kitchen counter so he can climb up and reach the sink. Put toys in the bath or kitchen sink. Use things that sink and things that float. Pour, splash, fill, and empty containers. Use a funnel. Use bubble bath or food colouring. Use warm water and cool water. Wash dishes, hands, dolls, clothes, and toys. Fill an empty wading pool.

When the child is in the bath or wading pool, attach a funnel to a small piece of lightweight plastic tubing. Wrap the tubing around the child's leg or trunk. Help the child pour water into the funnel. The child will be able to feel the water moving in the tubing and coming out at the end. He can move the tubing around his body. Old vacuum hoses and concertina-type dryer tubing can also be used and do not need a funnel. Use duct tape to tape over any wire ends in dryer tubing.

Fill balloons with water – a fun way to play ball on a hot day. A balloon filled with water can also be frozen and provide an ice ball to roll. Find puddles outside. Jump and splash in them.

Another favourite activity is to place the child in a wading pool or large shower stall. Squeeze a little honey, syrup, or liquid soap on the child's shoulder, back, or arm. As the liquid runs slowly down his body, encourage him to identify what part of the body he feels the liquid on. If honey or syrup is used, the child can enjoy licking his fingers and then being hosed clean. If liquid soap is used, the hosing will create bubbles – another enjoyable experience.

Sand play ideas. In a sandbox or on the beach, fill empty containers and scoop and dump. Cover body parts with sand. Search for toys hidden in the sand. Children need to learn early that sand is not for throwing. A child needs to be shown the boundary or edge of the sandbox. Add water to the sand to make hand- and footprints. Macaroni, cornmeal, or puffed wheat can be used in similar ways.

Hobbies. What is your child interested in? Can it be developed into a hobby? Is he interested in pets, cars, or stamp collections with interesting pictures, such as animals or ships? Stamp collections are especially good for partially sighted children with good central vision or myopic vision – they hold objects very close to the eye to see. Other collections can include buttons, pop cans, bottle tops, stones, books, tapes, or records.

Sounds. Visually impaired children rely on sensory cues to understand their environment. We often forget to identify these cues for them. Encourage your child to listen to different sounds. Tell the child what sound you hear or *what it is you think he is listening to.* If possible, let him touch and explore the source of the sound. Later you can ask the child to identify sounds. Here are some suggested sound-producing activities.

a Play the game of imitating sounds. You can play with your blind or visually impaired child. Take turns at making sounds, such as clapping, tapping, stamping, teeth chattering, blowing a raspberry, kissing, jumping, whistling, or snapping fingers.

b Teach your child to blow on his own hands, blow bubbles in the water, blow through a straw, blow out candles, blow into cylinders to make a noise, then try a whistle, recorder, or harmonica.

c Put a balloon up against the child's face. Pat the balloon gently to allow him to experience the sound and vibration. Encourage the child to do the same. Show him how to make a noise by putting his lips on the balloon and blowing.

d Stand on a quiet street. Listen for a car and show the child how to point to the car as it moves past you.

e Record some sounds and then have a quiz game. You could also record or play individual musical instruments and ask the child to identify them.

f Match sounds: put rice, stones, sugar, coins, etc., in empty yoghurt or pill containers. First tell the child what is making the sound. Ask him to find a specific sound and later to match two containers with the same sound.

Identifying smells. Identify smells for your child. If possible let him touch and explore the source. Later you can ask the child to identify smells, such as mustard, pepper, chocolate, beer, lemons, tea, coffee (in cup and on the breath), herbs and seasonings, baking, toothpaste, shampoo, shaving-cream, talcum powder, perfume, clean clothes, washing powder, lavender bag, hairdresser's shop, wet grass, mown grass, flowers, fir cones, fire, damp sawdust, pine needles, chlorine in swimming-pool, leather.

Use pillboxes or baby-food jars and put a different odorous item in each container, such as spice, food item, fragrant soap. These can be used as single items or in pairs for matching. Have the child identify and/or match with smells from other containers.

Identifying tastes. Identify different tastes of food. Give the child an opportunity to taste the same foods raw and cooked. Taste and label 'sweet,' 'sour,' 'salty,' etc. Introduce in a fun way small amounts of unpleasant tastes so the child learns what is not good to eat, e.g., sour milk, bruised fruit.

Textures and touch. Label textures: soft, hard, fuzzy, furry, rough, smooth, squishy, fluffy, scratchy, etc. Identify textures in everyday situations: furniture, food, clothes, fences, bricks, sidewalk, etc. Make

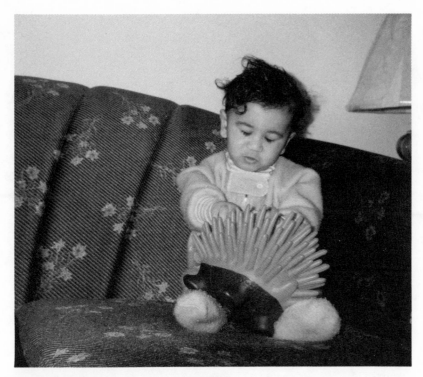

Tactile exploration.

a touch scrapbook of feathers, towelling, corrugated paper, sandpaper, etc. Use appropriate identification for textures, e.g., a smooth feather is a smooth feather, not a bird.

Differentiating between temperatures. Bring different temperatures to the child's attention. Check the weather daily. Experience snow, ice, rain, and sun. Bring snow indoors in a cup and/or bucket and feel it melt. An alternative would be to take ice out of the freezer into room temperature. Encourage the child to think of what clothes are worn in hot and cold weather. What would be comfortable to wear in both situations and why? Touch the walls and windows and comment on their temperature. Make connections between cold weather and a cold outside wall, or between the warmth of a stove and the wall beside it.

Show the child the differences in water temperature. Gradually let the water get warmer or colder by using both taps in a sink together.

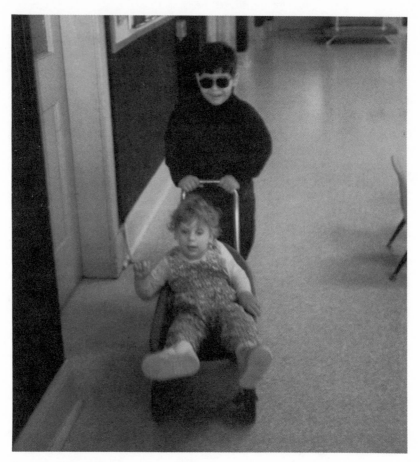

Imaginative and cooperative play.

Show your child how hot and steamy the bathroom is after someone
has had a shower.

Introduce your child to the warmth or cold of kitchen appliances
– the warmth of a stove (from a safe distance) and the chill of a
refrigerator. Touching the stove should be forbidden.

Pushing activities. Do activities that involve pushing. Activate a
humming top. Push a doll carriage, shopping cart, or other toys.
Push a door or drawer to close it. (Occasionally a door has to be
pushed to open it.) Push a chair under the table. (Remember, for the
blind child, it is only the seat part of the chair that is actually under

the table. You might like to ask the child what part of the chair is actually under the table.) Push a doorbell. Push an elevator button. Push a light switch. Push a flashlight switch.

Pulling activities. Do alternative pulling activities. Pull a toy on a string (often not enjoyed by blind children). Pull a drawer or door to open it. Pull a chair out from under the table. Pull pop beads apart. Pull in a tug-of-war game. Pull off socks and shoes. Pull to tear paper. Pull a Christmas cracker.

Sorting, matching, and comparing. Identify and match shapes, colours, smells, sounds, sizes, textures.

Make a home-made shape sorter. Make one round hole in the lid of a margarine container. Use a ball and then a cylinder to drop through the hole. Later as the child becomes more skilful, include other shapes, one at a time. Use different lids with appropriate cut-out. If you are using a commercially made shape sorter, at the beginning block off all the holes except the circle. Start with the circle and gradually include the other shapes.

Containers for sorting can include margarine containers, bowls, coffee tins, trays, drawers, egg cartons, muffin tins, or jewellery boxes. Things to sort can include bread tags, blocks, buttons, Smarties, raisins, tin-foil balls, paper-clips, clothes-pins, poker chips, pegs, ping-pong balls, spoons, forks, knives, cups, or coasters.

To start, give the child a bowl containing two very different items, e.g., paper-clips and blocks. Ask the child to hand you a block and then to find a paper-clip. When he can do this easily, ask the child to place the blocks in another container. As the child progresses, put several different items in one container and ask him to find and take out one specific item, and later sort them all into different containers.

At a more advanced level, use a tray to provide a boundary. You will need three containers for sorting items. Before placing anything on the tray, discuss the distinction between the right and left side of the tray. Then place a container on one side and identify left or right. Do the same on the other side. Practise by handing items to the child and asking him to place them in the right or left container. When the child can do this, place a container in the centre with two (later several) items and ask him to place certain items in the right-hand container and others in the left-hand container. Gradually increase the complexity until the child is sorting items that are very similar, e.g., pennies and dimes. (Given the opportunity, many blind children learn to be more tactile discriminating than their sighted peers.)

Place a number of different items along the top row of an egg carton. Place matching items together in the lid. Ask the child to find matching items from the lid and place them in the corresponding lower row.

Match different shapes. Draw a circle on a card, using a marker. A good contrast is black on white. Ask the child to put a corresponding sticky shape on the circle. Later draw two or three different shapes on the card and ask the child to stick on matching shapes. Stick four shapes on a card, three the same, one different. Ask the child to identify the odd one, then to draw or stick on an identical shape under or above the one that is different.

Threading activities. Items to thread: beads, hair rollers, bangles, thread spools, straws, buttons, toilet-paper rolls, paper-towel rolls, paper-clips, Lifesavers, cereal. To make and thread tin-foil balls, use a square piece of tin foil. Push threaded needle through the centre, then crumple tin foil to form a ball around the thread.

For threading, use wool, string (dip ends in nail polish or glue to make threading easier or wrap ends with tape), shoe or skate laces, pipe-cleaners, a small stick, or elastic used with a large, blunt wool needle.

Thread items in a simple pattern of specific shapes, colours, and sizes. Copy a pattern. Make a necklace.

Other items to thread are nuts and bolts. Start with large ones and progress to small ones. When using nuts and bolts, line them up according to size, using the edge of a tray to keep the line straight. Always work from left to right. To make threading easier, especially for multihandicapped children, long bolts can be imbedded in a shallow tin into which you have poured plaster of Paris. Push the bolts head side down into the plaster of Paris as it begins to harden. This secures the bolts.

Drawing activities. For the partially sighted child use good contrasts, e.g., black felt pen or red crayon on white paper, white chalk on black board. For the totally blind child use wax crayons and a mesh board. To make a mesh board, place metal window screening taut over a wooden board or bulletin-board and staple the mesh firmly in place. Any rough edges can then be covered with plastic tape. (Do not use fibreglass screening, as it stretches.) Place paper on the board. If a bulletin-board is used, the paper can be kept in place with thumbtacks. Allow the child to scribble at random and look at or feel the lines he has made. Show the child how to draw straight lines, a circle, and a square. Encourage him to look at or feel what he has done.

For small blind children use geometric shapes, not three-dimensional representations.

Gross-motor activities

Obstacle course. Explore the obstacle course with a visually impaired child, then talk him through it. A sample indoor obstacle course starts under a chair, over a stool, short tunnel made of a large box, under cushions, under table, in between two pieces of furniture, up the stairs, somersault on the bed. An outdoor obstacle course can start under the picnic table, up the climbing frame, down the slide, through a tunnel made of a large box, through the sandbox, over a sturdy chair.

Three-legged walk. The child and adult stand side by side. Tie the child's left ankle and the adult's right ankle together with a scarf. Walk together. Let two children try it together. It's lots of fun and later it can be a race against another team. Team a blind child with a sighted one.

Play equipment. Have some play equipment in your yard to attract other children and encourage them to interact with your visually impaired child.

Errands. Ask your child to do errands to practise his skills – for example, 'Please take the newspaper to Daddy'; 'Please take your bib to the table'; 'Please bring me the red book from the coffee-table'; 'Can you put this soap on the bathroom counter?' Have your child put away shopping items.

A fun indoor activity. Children can pull each other on mats or towels on the polished floor.

Roller skating. Roller skate on the carpet with small children. They really enjoy pushing skates backwards and forwards. Allow children to play with the roller skates before encouraging them to wear them.

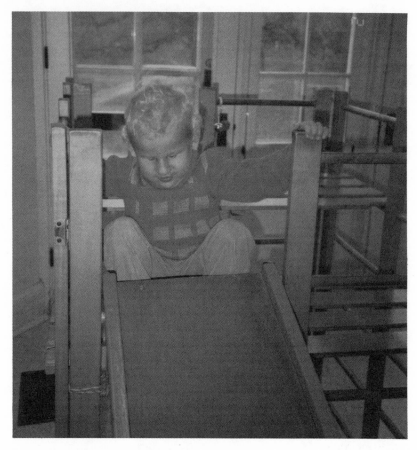

Fun on the climbing frame and slide.

Exploration replaces observation. A chair to hold onto is helpful. He may need your help, as roller skates make the child move faster than he is used to. Speed is a great experience for him! Arrange a clear space. Let him hold your hand, one side of a hoop, or fix up a rope that he can hold onto and move along back and forth until he is competent enough to skate independently. When the child is able to balance and move on the carpet, try a different surface – grass or a wooden floor. Even totally blind children can become skilled at roller skating, as well as ice skating.

Hoops. You can use a hoop for your child to hold on to when learning to walk. He holds one side and you hold the other. This is fun even after the child is walking well. He can run, jump, skip, or roller skate with it. Put a bell on the hoop for added interest.

Hoops give the idea of a big circle. Put a tactile marker on the hoop, have the child touch the marker and walk around the hoop until he finds the marker again. You can also let the visually impaired child lie in the hoop, feet touching one side, hands the other. Use the tactile marker again, slowly move the hoop round so the child feels the movement until the marker is back in his hand. To reinforce the idea, have a group of children sitting around the hoop. Let the visually impaired child sit in the hoop and reach in all directions to find the hoop and the other children.

Visually impaired children often have difficulty sharing space. Let one or two children sit inside the hoop with the visually impaired child and play a game. The first game may need to be played with only one other child. An adult claps once and the first child jumps or steps into the hoop; the adult claps twice and the second child jumps or steps into the hoop. The adult stamps and both children move out of the hoop. Vary this game and gradually increase the amount of time the children are in the hoop. When children are comfortable with sharing space, play a game of seeing how many children can squeeze into the hoop. Count children by claps as they go in and by numbers as they come out.

Stilts. Walk on coffee-tin stilts. Use two empty coffee tins with plastic lids. Punch a hole about an inch from the bottom on each side. Thread a rope or clothes-line through the holes to the height of the child's hands when standing on tins. Tie with a knot inside the tin. The secret of walking on these stilts is to keep the rope taut. Walk on carpet. Start with the child leaning against the wall. This is a difficult activity for most blind children.

Books. Visually impaired children enjoy stories and books. Reading with infants, toddlers, and preschoolers has many benefits. We believe that young children also need books available at all times where they can reach, select, and look at them by themselves or with a friend. These books need to be sturdy as they will receive a lot of rough use. Board books are durable and usually small and light enough in weight for the child to hold. Small photo albums also have the same advantages and pages are easily manipulated by the child. The contents and topics can change from time to time. Suggestions for the books: simple pictures that you have drawn, clear photographs, uncluttered magazine pictures of animals, babies, toys, and household items. You can also use coloured paper on some pages and geometric shapes and patterns on others.

Pictures should be clear, colourful, and provide a good contrast to a plain background. Label pictures with one word, then progress to simple sentences, and later develop an appropriate story.

Subject-matter should relate to the child's experiences, such as baby's routine times, household activities, animals, car rides, feelings, friends and family, food, maybe the policeman on horseback he met on the morning walk.

Tactile books. You can make your own books out of cloth, cardboard, and binder rings, or use photo albums. Pages can also be made of cloth with metal grommets to be used in a binder. Attach to the pages familiar articles, such as a real toothbrush, comb, crayons, barrettes, socks, small bell, face-cloth, rattle, or squeaker; some textures, such as ribbon, corduroy, denim, velvet, wool, leather, cotton, carpet, deck-chair material, towelling, wallpaper, fake fur, blanket, sheet, wood, plastic, string, straw, feathers, corrugated paper, cotton batting, paper, sandpaper, elastic bands.

For blind preschool children do not use cut-out representations, such as a cut-out horse or rabbit. This can cause confusion in developing concepts at the preschool level. If a blind child is to understand thermoform raised pictures or other tactile representations, he will need to be taught. First he must be able to recognize the concrete object, e.g., a button, small spoon, or nail; then the representation and the actual object should be teamed together. As the child matures and understands the idea of representation, he may be able to recognize larger representations of people and animals.

Make a texture book. Cut strips of fabric approximately 12 inches by 6 inches (30.5 cm by 15 cm). Fold in half, the right sides together. Stitch the two sides. Turn inside out and press. If attaching items to the pages, do this before folding and stitching sides.

Make five more pages as above, using different textures. Place all the pages together. Using 2-inch (5 cm) cloth tape, cut to the length of the open side. Place pages on one-half of tape. Fold tape and pin in place. Sew together to bind the pages. Make 4-in (10 cm) square patches for the child to match with pages. Follow the directions for

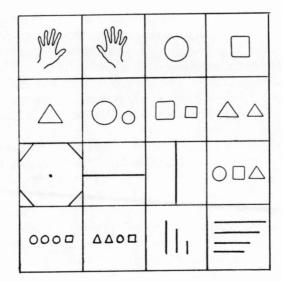

Sixteen suggested pages for a home-made tactile book.

pages, but sew all four sides. Make a cover for the book with a pocket to store the patches safely.

Make a book out of cloth. Sew on each page a pocket fastened with a different fastening, for example, Velcro, domes, hook-and-eye, zipper, button, buckle. Put a surprise in each pocket to encourage opening. Add a tactile marker to indicate the top right-hand corner of each page (button or a small piece of matchstick). If the pockets are bulky, use the grommet-and-binder method.

Make a book out of cloth or card. Divide each page into squares (see diagram) by gluing on string, wool, or popsicle sticks. Make shapes from felt, sandpaper, plastic, etc. The child can identify hands, right, left, specific fingers, shapes, big, small, short, long, same or different – there are numerous combinations. Using candies, buttons, or poker chips, the child can place one or more items in corners, centre, above, below, on, or at the end of lines. You could have one page with the soft side of Velcro lines stitched or glued on, and a few detachable shapes with the corresponding rough side of the Velcro attached. This would allow for changing positions of the various shapes and would add interest and new challenges. This kind of book is good at the kindergarten level.

Housekeeping activities that provide fun learning experiences.
Visually impaired children need many repeated experiences with
appropriate language to help them learn about their world. Whenever possible, include them in daily household routines. How much
they participate will, or course, depend on their age and ability and
your time and energy. Even a toddler can accompany you as you
perform tasks and participate by helping to carry socks and put them
in the washer.

Sighted children gain information by watching activities and learning can take place incidentally. Through this observation, they are
frequently motivated to want to help. The visually impaired child is
often not aware of the activity and the many steps involved. Even
though he may be with you, unless you take the time to explain and
encourage him to participate, he will miss these incidental learning
experiences. Gradually increase the child's participation in these
activities. *Do not feel overwhelmed. It is not necessary to do these things
every time.*

The laundry cycle. Let the child put his dirty clothes in the laundry
basket; help you carry the things to the laundry room; take the laundry to the washer, sort out the clothes and the household linen; help
put the clothes in the washer; turn on the washer, listen, feel the
vibration; take clothes out of the washer; put the clothes in the dryer;
turn on the dryer; wait for the cycle to finish. The waiting period
helps the child understand about time and he'll need some activities
to fill in that time. Take the clothes out of the dryer; shake and
fold, sort, name items, identify what they are, what they are used
for, and whose they are. Put in the laundry basket. Put items to be
ironed on the ironing-board. Let the child feel the crumpled clothes
and then later the smooth clothes. Talk about ironing; let the child
feel the warm clothes after the iron has been over them. The child
may enjoy a toy ironing-board at this point (beginning role-play). Put
clothes away. Let the child help find the clothes to wear next day,
finding them in the drawer or cupboard where they were put after
laundering.

Shopping. Take the child with you to the supermarket, explore items
on shelves. Experience hot and cold, smells, sounds; put items in the
cart; take items out of the cart and put them on the cashier's counter
(explore conveyor belt); talk to cashier; pay for groceries; give the
child a specific coin to give the cashier, so that he becomes familiar

with different coins; put items into bags and into buggy; carry home or to the car; carry from the car to the kitchen (the child can experience heavy and lightweight items). Put items on the kitchen shelves. Later encourage him to find the same items when needed.

Taking out garbage. Let the child put banana skin, broken toys, etc., in garbage and put appropriate bottles and cans in the recycle container; help tie up the garbage bags; take them outside or to the garbage chute; help fit a clean garbage bag into the empty holder. Meet the garbage truck, talk to the driver, watch or listen to the garbage man throwing the garbage bag into the truck.

Cleaning. Let the child help with vacuuming, or tell the child what you are doing when you are cleaning around the house. You can put a dust pile on the floor, allow the child to feel it, and then sweep it up into the dustpan. Let the child explore the vacuum after the canister is emptied. Tear up newspaper into small pieces and crumple (good for fine-muscle activity). Place pieces into a heavy container, for example, a large saucepan. Let the child turn on the machine and vacuum up the paper. Open canister and find paper. Empty into the garbage.

Dishwashing. Take a dirty dish or cup to the sink; put on an apron; help to pull a chair up to the counter so that the child can reach the sink. Turn on the taps, get the right temperature of water, add detergent, wash, and identify dishes. Put on the counter to drain, empty the sink, dry the dishes. Put away in the cupboard. Put dishes in the dishwasher, add detergent, note the fragrance, take out the dishes, and put them away in the cupboard. Discuss dirty dishes, clean dishes, and hot water.

Helping plant beans and watching them grow. Use an empty jam jar and line the inside of the jar with a paper towel or blotting paper. Put two or three beans between the paper and the glass jar. Dampen the paper and keep it damp by regular watering. A small amount of water in the bottom of the jar is absorbed by the paper. Watch beans sprout, both roots and shoots.

Cooking. Let your child be in the kitchen with you whenever possible. Place frequently used, safe utensils within his reach. As you need them, ask him to give you measuring-spoons, rolling-pin, etc.

Describe what you are doing. Let him help wash vegetables as you prepare dinner, maybe peel potatoes or tear the lettuce. He could help scoop ice-cream. Discuss where it is kept. Why is it cold and hard? Observe it melt in the warm kitchen. Here are some easy food preparation steps that your child can participate in:

- Freeze juice in paper cups with popsicle sticks for handles.
- Make popcorn. Let the child listen to the popping noise and smell the aroma, then experiment with different tastes. Add salt, butter, syrup, honey, or cheese.
- Make KoolAid or Freshie. Take juice out of the fridge and pour into cups.
- Bake apples or potatoes.
- Help make sandwiches. Have the child put precut cheese or meat on bread. Later show him how to spread butter, jam, and peanut butter on bread. Begin by using a slice of frozen bread – it is firmer and easier to handle. Make sure the butter or spread is soft. A narrow, flexible, short-handled spatula sometimes makes spreading easier.
- Wash celery and cut into 3-inch (7.5 cm) pieces. Fill with cheese spread or grated cheese and mayonnaise or peanut butter.
- Later with experience, the child can learn to choose his own lunch. Begin with two choices and gradually increase the choices.
- For quick, no-flour peanut butter cookies, you will need:

1 cup	crunchy peanut butter	250 mL
1	egg	1
1 cup	sugar	250 mL
$\frac{1}{2}$ tsp	vanilla	2 mL

Mix all ingredients in a bowl. Encourage the child to use his hands to form the dough. Have a damp sponge available for wiping hands. Roll the mixture into small, walnut-size balls. Place on an ungreased baking sheet. Flatten with a fork. Bake at 350°F (180°C) for 7–10 minutes. As options to the basic recipe, add nuts, raisins, chocolate, or caramel chips. Or use the basic recipe, but indent cookie with thumb before baking and fill with a small amount of jam.

- Allow the child to help with clean-up after cooking.
- Sit at the table and eat the freshly baked cookies. Have the child put cookies on the plate and pass it around to others. Teach the child to take one cookie off the plate.

Help bathe the baby. Bathing the baby gives lots of fun and opportunity for touching and naming body parts, comparing size, being gentle, etc. After bathing the baby, encourage imaginative play, such as bathing a doll.

Taking care of pets. Take the dog for a walk. Even if the child is in the stroller, he should be made aware that the dog is with you. He may like to help hold the lead. The child can help with feeding, putting out food for the dog, cat, hamster, or turtle. This way he learns what animals eat. He can watch and listen to the animals eating and drinking, brush the dog's hair, stroke the animal, find body parts, and compare. For fun, children may like to try to lap up water from a dish on the floor as a dog does, but they should be told not to experiment using the dog's dish.

Having a pet increases your child's experiences. A pet is always a responsibility and often a long-term one. Unless you enjoy animals and want one for its own sake, do not buy one. Instead go to pet shops, petting zoos, or visit friends who have pets. Repeat these experiences.

A pet is not a guide-dog for your child. A guide-dog is a well-trained working dog. No one is eligible to have a guide-dog until he is a young adult and has good mobility skills. The dog and potential owner are matched for compatibility and learn to work together as a team. The visually impaired person is responsible for the dog's care. Many visually impaired animal lovers prefer other means of mobility assistance, such as a cane.

Handyman jobs. Many little boys and girls like to help parents mend and make things, examining the tools, twisting and turning screws, sanding wood, hitting nails with a hammer, helping to saw, hand over hand.

Helping Mum or Dad fill the gas tank. Explain that cars need gas to run. Get out of the car at the gas station and let the child explore the pump. The child can help open the tank and put the nozzle in. Partially sighted children can be shown the numbers moving quickly on the gas pumps. Close the tank and return pipe to pump.

Helping wash the car. Have the child assist the adults in washing the car by giving him specific parts to wash, such as the hub-caps or the ashtray. Empty the ashtrays; polish the lights; dust the dashboard;

vacuum the back seat. Allow the child to help you collect the cleaning equipment needed and replace it afterwards.

Car rides. Take time to talk about the car and give the child lots of opportunities to explore the vehicle. When asked, 'What is a car?' one little girl replied, 'A chesterfield that moves,' which described her experience. Let your child find the wheels, the steering-wheel, the windshield wipers, and the button or knob that activates them. Allow him to open and close the doors and trunk, and explore the glove compartment, front and back seats, indicator lights, trunk, etc.

When going for a ride in the car, talk about your destination, the route, the sounds, the smells, the bumps, driving fast, driving slowly, driving straight, turning corners, observing traffic-lights and stop signs. If you are going on a long trip, take some toys to play with and some old handbags with zippers that he can put the toys in. String a line from door to door and attach items to the string with curtain rings or metal rings. Include magnetic boards with shapes and letters, suction cups on window and dashboard, a textured blanket, and tapes of favourite sounds. Plan a surprise: food, a special song, or a special stop on the way.

Places to visit. Petting zoo, supermarket, leather clothing store, butcher store, bread shop, toy store, local variety store, farm, apple orchard, airport, garden, beach, doctor's office, dentist's office, restaurant, stables, friends' and relatives' homes (maybe staying with them overnight), playground, shopping mall, park, bus depot, train station, marina, or car-park. Repeated visits will be necessary. Focus on a different aspect of each place every time.

Ways to travel. Give your child opportunities to experience different modes of travel, e.g., subway, car, train, plane, bus, bicycle, tractor, truck.

Group activities to get involved in. Ice skating, bowling, swimming, kindergym, jogging with parents, roller skating, horseback riding, tobogganing.

Have a friend over for juice and cookies. Before the visit role-play, practice, and preparation will be necessary.

Ideas for a child in hospital. Take a notice into the hospital with you to attach to his crib or bed. Write with permanent felt pen on a card. The message could read: 'My name is Joey. I can't see you. Please tell me who you are and what you are going to do.' Through vision, sighted children can usually anticipate whether an experience will be pleasant or unpleasant. A visually impaired child who cannot anticipate experiences may fear all physical contact if he was not warned whenever something unpleasant was about to happen to him.

Visually impaired children always need to be prepared for anything unpleasant or painful, such as a gentle pull on the right ear lobe, accompanied by the word 'hurt' before an injection is given or blood is taken. We suggest that you take a number of sticky labels on which you have written the warning sign you would like the hospital personnel to use. Give these to your child's special nurse or the head nurse and ask her to attach them to the appropriate files.

SIX

Action Songs and Chants

Songs marked with an asterisk (*) are especially suitable for infants as they are short, simple, and repetitive.

1. Mrs Murphy Had a Band

(Sung to the tune of 'Old McDonald Had a Farm')

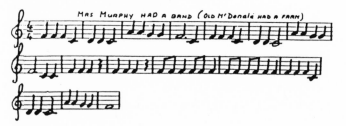

Mrs Murphy had a band
E-I-E-I-O
And in this band she had
A drum
E-I-E-I-O
With a bang bang here
And a bang bang there
Here a bang, there a bang
Everywhere a bang bang
Mrs Murphy had a band
E-I-E-I-O

Repeat with:
- A rattle
  With a rattle rattle here, etc.
- A bell
  with a ding ding here, etc.
- A shaker
  With a shake shake here, etc.
- A tambourine
  With a bang ting here, etc.
- Two sticks
  With a click click here, etc.
- Two lids
  With a crash crash here, etc.
- A whistle
  With a blow blow here, etc.
- A mouth organ
  With a woo woo here, etc.
- Two hands
  With a clap clap here, etc.

Metal buckets and large ice-cream containers make good drums. Shampoo, detergent, and yoghurt containers filled with beans, rice, macaroni, and pebbles make good shakers.

For the multihandicapped child who has difficulty holding items, the bells can be attached to elastic and placed on foot or wrist. Attach any item to his clothing closest to the limb he can move most easily. Give him time and encourage him to try on his own, however limited his movements may be.

*2. Here We Go Round the . . .

The old favourite 'Here We Go Round the Mulberry Bush' can become more meaningful if you change a few words.

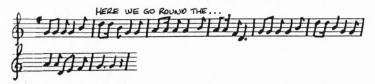

Here we go round the coffee-table
Coffee-table, coffee-table

Here we go round the coffee-table
With Mummy (Daddy) in the morning

This is the way we touch our toes
Touch our toes, touch our toes
This is the way we touch our toes
With Mummy (Daddy) in the morning

Repeat with:
• brush our hair
• wash our hands
• change your diaper
• stand up tall

3. One Little, Two Little, Three Little Fingers

(Sung to the tune of 'Ten Little Indians')

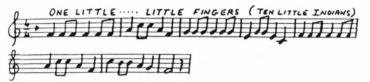

One little, two little, three little fingers
Four little, five little, six little fingers
Seven little, eight little, nine little fingers
Ten little fingers together.

The following verses are designed to help develop the concept of thumb and fingers.

On my right hand I've got four fingers
On my right hand I've got four fingers
On my right hand I've got four fingers
One, two, three, and four

On my left hand I've got four fingers
On my left hand I've got four fingers
On my left hand I've got four fingers
Eight little fingers together

On my right hand I have one thumb
On my left hand I have one thumb
On my right hand I have one thumb
Wiggle both thumbs together

Clap your hands and wiggle your fingers
Clap your hands and wiggle your fingers
Clap your hands and wiggle your fingers
Clap clap clap clap clap

4. Rhyming Nonsense Chants

Clap and chant some easy nonsense rhymes to introduce a variety of
vowels and consonants.

    a) Cat, bat, hat, rat, all sitting on the mat.
    b) Pitter-patter, pitter-patter, listen to the rain.
    c) Hickety, pickety, poppety pet, splash in the puddles and all get wet.
    d) Wiggles and whirls and twiggles and twirls, some are boys and some
       are girls.

5. Clap the Beat of Different Words

*Mummy, Daddy, Alison, John, Margareta, apple, banana, pomegranate,
Cheerios, milk, sweater, socks.*

6. Head and Shoulders

(Sung to the tune of 'London Bridge')

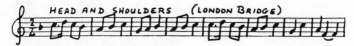

Head and shoulders, knees and toes
Knees and toes, knees and toes
Head and shoulders, knees and toes
Eyes, ears, mouth (or chin), and nose

You can use different body parts – hip and lip, palm and arm, thumb
and bum, to give you rhyming words.

7. Back and Forth and Back and Forth

(Sung to the tune of 'Row, Row, Row Your Boat')

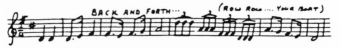

Back and forth and back and forth, nearly touching the floor.
Merrily, merrily, merrily, merrily, now we'll do it some more.
Back and forth, and back and forth, backs right to the floor [sing slowly]
Merrily, merrily, merrily, merrily, shall we do it once more

*8. If You're Happy and You Know It

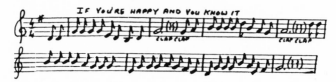

If you're happy and you know it
Clap your hands
If you're happy and you know it
Clap your hands
If you're happy and you know it
And you really want to show it
If you're happy and you know it
Clap your hands

Other verses could be:

- Touch your knees
- Snap your fingers
- Stamp your feet
- Jump up and down
- Touch your toes
- Shout hurray

9. Hokey Pokey

The words 'forward' and 'backward' replace the 'in' and 'out' of the original song, which may be confusing to some young blind children who do not see the circle.

You put your right foot forward [or in front]
You put your right foot backward [or behind]
You put your right foot forward
And you shake it all about
You do the hokey pokey
And you turn around
That's what it's all about – hey!

Oh, the hokey pokey
Oh, the hokey pokey
Oh, the hokey pokey
And that's what it's all about

10. Running on the Spot Chant

To understand running on the spot or in a confined space, allow children to run inside hula hoops.

I am running on the spot
An exercise I like a lot
On my toes I can run
Up and down, this is fun
Round and round and round I go
Still on the same spot, did you know
Swinging my arms to and fro
Round and round again I go
Running, running on this spot
Soon I'll be both tired and hot
Huffing, puffing, now I'm slowing
But I think I must keep going
Come and run along with me
It is fun, you will see

11. Skipping Song

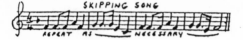

Hop with my right foot
Step with my left foot
Hop with my left foot (slowly moving forward)
Step with my right foot

Repeat once, or continue singing slowly, keeping the beat until the child moves easily in rhythm. Sing a little faster, keeping good rhythm:

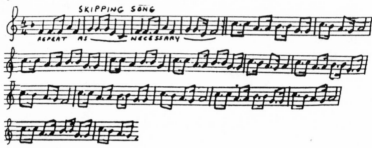

Hop and step and hop and step
Singing as we go
Hop and step and hop and step
Knees up high, feet down low
Hop and step and hop and step
Skipping's fun, you know
Hop and step and hop and step
It's nearly time to slow

Skipping, skipping, skipping, skipping
Singing as we go
Skipping, skipping, skipping, skipping
Skipping to and fro
Skipping, skipping, skipping, skipping
Now it's time to slow

Finish by saying, 'And stop,' or repeat the beginning or second and third verses.

12. Sunday School Song

Point to body parts as the song is sung.

Two little eyes to look to God
Two little ears to hear his word
Two little feet to walk in his ways
Two little lips to sing his praise
Two little hands to do his will
One little heart to love him still

SEVEN

Games and Crafts

The following games include well-known old favourites, as well as some new ones, with adaptations for the visually impaired child. Games need to be thought through carefully and attention given to details. If the visually impaired child is to understand the rules and progression of the game, the instructions should be precise, particularly in a group situation. These games can be played with an individual child, a group of visually impaired children, or a group that includes a visually impaired child. Your choice of games will, of course, depend on the children's developmental level and experiences. You may be able to think of other variations to suit the child or children in your care.

Musical Chairs

Chairs are lined up facing alternate directions, with one chair fewer than the number of players. Children run, walk, or dance around the chairs until the music stops. Then they must find a seat. The one who does not find a chair is out. One chair is removed. When the music starts again, children walk around chairs. Repeat until one chair remains. The child who sits on this one when the music stops is the winner.

You may need to play this game with only two or three children at first. Set up the chairs and allow the visually impaired children to explore the arrangement. For very young children have one chair for each child, then the game is for everyone to find a seat when the music stops. All children may like to take a turn at providing the music – for example, switching on and off the tape machine, banging the drum or tambourine, shaking bells.

Drumbeat or Musical Stepping-Stones

For developing tactile discrimination, make stepping-stones of different textures by sticking fabrics, sandpaper, corrugated paper, fake fur, florist's paper, carpet pieces, sponge, plastic, etc., onto foot-size cards. Spread the completed cards around the floor – one for each child. Have the children go barefoot and dance around the room. When the music stops, they stand on a fabric stone. The teacher then quizzes one or more of the children about the fabric they are standing on: e.g., 'What does your stone feel like? Is it soft, bumpy, or rough?' If there is a totally blind child in the class, arrange the stepping-stones close to a wall or in some kind of order to make them easier to locate. If the blind child still has difficulty, allow another child or the teacher to partner him.

Musical Circle Games

a The children sit on the floor in a circle. Place a box containing common articles in the centre, such as a spinning-top, toy phone, hat, crayons, rattle, towel, zipper, spoon, shoe. When the music starts, the children pass around a beanbag. Make sure the visually impaired child knows who is on either side of him and which way the beanbag is moving around the circle. When the music stops, the child with the beanbag goes to the centre of the circle to find an article in the box. He names what he finds and talks about how the article is used or demonstrates its use. If the child participates he receives a clap from the group. Remember, the visually impaired child will need verbal information to understand the actions of the child in the centre.

A variation on this for younger or physically handicapped children is to have everyone dance or clap until the music stops. They sit down and the adult chooses a child to go to the box. If there is a non-ambulatory child in the group, the teacher takes the box to each child. An alternative to a beanbag could be a ball with a bell inside, which could be made from a 'Nerf' (foam) ball by cutting it open and putting a bell in the centre, and then sticking the ball together.

b The children sit on the floor in a circle. Someone plays a musical instrument or a tape recorder. Each time the music stops, a direction is given. Suggested directions: all the boys stand up and stamp; all the girls stand up and jump; all the adults stand up and clap; all the children stand up and turn around; everybody joins hands in a circle and walks; etc. Or the directions could relate to clothing: e.g., everyone wearing long pants, stand up and clap; children wearing shoes or sandals/glasses/a dress/necklace, stand up and jump, skip, shake, roll, etc.

c The teacher hides a familiar article in a bag. As the children sing the song below, it is passed around the circle. After the word 'thing,' use the name of the child holding the bag. This child feels the object inside the bag and guesses what it is. After making a guess, the child pulls it out of the bag for all to see. Everyone claps while the teacher puts another article in the bag. The game begins again from a different place in the circle. If there are only a few children, they could sit around a hula hoop. Compare a ring for a finger to a hula hoop, which is like a large ring that can fit over a whole body or a small group of children. A music circle is like a ring of people.

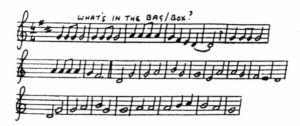

What's in the bag, what's in the bag
What's in the bag today today
What's in the bag, what's in the bag
What's in the bag today
Pass it round the people ring
I wonder what is in this thing
(Child's name) it's your turn to play
Tell us what's in the bag today

Body Positions

The children walk around the room or area while music is being played. (It helps the visually impaired child if boundaries are made clear.) Each time the music stops, tell the children to: 'Make yourself tall, or small, higher than me, close to the floor, roll into a ball,' etc.

Find the Spot

This musical game can be played indoors or outdoors. The children can dance, jump, or run when the music is heard. If played outside, use a drum, rattles, bells, or clapping. When the music stops the children stop and follow the teacher's direction, which could be to stand in the sun or the shade, stand in a draft or on carpet, wood, linoleum, tile, grass, or gravel. It will be easier if you first familiarize the visually impaired child with the area. Some totally blind children (without light perception) may be able to find the warm spot in the sunshine, while others will need a partner to help them.

Hot Potato

Sing this song to the tune of 'London Bridge.'

> Hot potato, pass it on, pass it on, pass it on
> Hot potato, pass it on
> Get ready for the hot potato

All the children sit in a circle. When singing begins, they quickly pass around the 'hot potato.' (You could use a beanbag with a bell attached to help the visually impaired child follow the movement of the hot potato.) When the song ends, the child who is holding the hot potato is out. This continues until one child – the winner – is left.

It is sometimes more fun for young children if the child holding the hot potato is allowed to stay in the game with just a comment, e.g., 'Joan has the hot potato this time. Let's start the song, pass it on quickly.' It will be helpful for the blind or visually impaired child to play a one-to-one game with an adult first to practise passing.

Talk about a real hot potato and the pretend one. An alternative is to fill a balloon with water and freeze it. Pass the frozen ball around the circle. Change 'hot potato' to 'icy ball' in the song.

Pass the Shoe

The children sit in a circle. Each child takes off one shoe. Pass the shoes around the circle once or twice until each child finds his own again. As the shoes are passed around, the children could say, 'Not my shoe, not my shoe,' and then, 'This is my shoe.' Control the speed of passing by calling 'Pass' to provide enough time for the visually impaired child to feel each shoe.

Boxes

Have a collection of boxes of various sizes with lids. The largest should be one big enough for the child to climb into. The smallest could be small enough to fit into the child's hand. Fit the boxes one inside the other. Ask the child to remove the first lid and lift out the next box. Continue until he reaches the smallest box, in which you have hidden a special surprise. Other boxes could also have little surprises for encouragement. Later the child can match the lids to the boxes, and also climb in and out of the bigger boxes. The child could also be encouraged to step from one box lid to another (stepping-stones), or to stack and knock them over. For added enjoyment, the boxes could be covered with textured material. For durability, strengthen boxes with masking or duct tape before covering.

To encourage other movements, use rhymes such as:

Jack-in-the-box
Sits so still.
Won't you come out?
Yes, I will!

Have the child crouch down inside a large cardboard box and jump up at the end of the rhyme. To make it more fun, put newspaper over the top of the box so the child will feel and hear the paper as he jumps up.

Simon Says

For very young children, this can begin as 'Mummy says.' Give a few very simple directions: for example, 'Touch your mouth,' 'Tickle your tummy,' then end with 'Give me a hug.'

For a group game, the leader gives directions and the children only respond if the preface 'Simon says' is used. If a child follows a direction when 'Simon says' is *not* used, the child is out. The game continues until only one child is left in the game – the winner. Begin with simple one-step directions given slowly. Gradually increase speed. An opportunity to play this game individually is a good idea before a child joins a group.

This is a fun game for teaching less familiar body parts and for finding out what a child knows about his body. When playing this game in a group of older children, include more complicated directions: for example, 'Touch any body part below your knee,' 'Any part above your waist,' 'Put your hands on your throat/collarbone/ankle/hips,' 'Put your middle/baby finger on your nose/eyebrow,' 'Put your thumb on your heel/big toe,' 'Fold your arms and stamp your feet,' 'Lie on your right side,' 'Take a step forwards/backwards/to the right/left,' 'Lie on your back and lift your head,' 'Bend your knees.'

I Spy

This can be played with visually impaired children. As for the sighted child, clues need to be geared to the visually impaired child's level of ability. Remember, the visually impaired child will need to move around in search of the object. It will not be a sedentary game unless the objects are confined to the table or pictures in a book. Set some height and distance boundaries at the beginning of the game if sighted and visually impaired children play together: e.g., not higher than ... or farther than ...

The totally blind child can also play this game, but it becomes more a game of hide-and-seek. Use clues that require the use of other senses: for example, 'I am thinking of a special toy that makes a squeaky sound. Can you find it?' This game is probably best played on an individual basis or with two or three blind children.

Hide-and-Seek

In Hide-and-Seek one person closes his eyes and counts to an agreed-upon number to give other players time to hide. That person then tries to find everyone. The first person found is the next seeker. There are many variations on this old favourite that can be played with visually impaired preschoolers. Hide-and-Seek provides fun experiences for practising exploring and searching techniques, listening and language skills, mobility skills, ear/hand and eye/hand coordination. It also provides opportunities to introduce and develop understanding of concepts.

When the blind or visually impaired child plays Hide-and-Seek with one or two sighted children, it can heighten everyone's awareness of the fact that the blind or visually impaired child 'sees' differently. Be prepared for questions. Some variations:

Hide an object. Ask the child to find the object. Then give the child a turn to hide it and you try to find it. Where you hide the object and the clues you give will depend on the needs of the child and his level of skill. Very small children can play this too and love to search for a toy hidden in their own clothing or on the adults. Objects can be totally or partially hidden. Objects can have a sound – continuous or intermittent. Give praise when the object is found. The child will most likely hide the object for you to find in the place he found it. This is okay at first. With experience, he will begin to think of his own hiding places. If not, he may need assistance from another person to help him hide it.

When the child is becoming competent at seeking, he may like some competition – for example, finding the object before the kitchen timer buzzes. If this form of Hide-and-Seek is played with a visually impaired child and a sighted child, you may need to hide one object for each child, or you may have to think out your clues more carefully so that both children have an equal chance to be the first to find the object. Sometimes, whispering clues in the ear is fun and the clues need not be identical. Another way to play this game is to explain to the child, 'As you get closer to the hidden object, I will clap my hands, and if you move away, I will stamp my feet,' or 'I will sing loudly as you get closer and quietly if you move away.'

Hide a person. When you hide from a blind or visually impaired child, you can make a continuous sound (sing quietly), or an intermittent sound (occasionally clicking your tongue), or just call 'Ready' when you are hidden. Again, what you say or do will depend on the child's visual ability and level of skill. Reward the finding with a hug or exclamation of surprise and start again. Give your child clues before you hide. They may be general or specific. For example: 'I am going to hide in the bathroom'; 'I am going to be hiding behind a chair in this room'; 'I am going to be lying down on something in the bedroom'; 'I am going to hide upstairs.'

When the blind or visually impaired child is hiding from you or a sighted friend, he needs to learn that to be hidden, he must be completely behind or under something. If both children are hiding from the adult, they should hide together. 'Behind' is a difficult concept. The hiding child may hide behind an object, but as the seeker moves, the child may no longer be behind the object.

Locating the Music Box

This game is suitable for nursery school level through teens. It can also be played with older sighted children who are blindfolded. Use a music box or timer. Start by winding up the music box fully or putting the timer on for a longer period. The children try to find the music box or timer before the sound stops.

Reduce the length of time as the children become more skilful. Place the music box high, low, or at waist level. In time, it can also be placed inside, under, or behind things. One position the children find most difficult is when the box is placed on a centre shelf that is narrower than the top shelf, say, of a bookcase. The child reaches up and down, but frequently misses the centre shelf.

Moving in Pairs

This is excellent for giving a blind child the feel of another's body moving, while he does the same action. Small sighted children enjoy this too. Have one child stand behind the other and lightly hold the waist of the person in front. The adult then instructs the children to bend forward or sideways; to step forward with right foot and back again onto left foot in a rocking motion. Teach very simple steps in rhythmic movements and do them to music. Blind children should be given opportunities to be in front and behind.

Do simple actions with children side by side, arms around each other's waist. Walk forwards, backwards, or round in a circle as instructed. Facing each other, do actions such as stamping, tapping, clapping right hands together, left hands together, in sequence, etc.

Statues

Children move around the room to the sound of music or a drum beat. The adult calls out instructions that encourage body movement, such as waving arms, swaying from the waist, turning around and around, running on tiptoes, taking big steps, and stamping along. When the music stops, the children freeze into statues in whatever position they are in until the music starts again. If anyone moves before the music starts, he is out.

Follow-the-Leader

A leader is chosen. The children follow the leader around the room or yard and do exactly as he does. Each child is given a chance to be leader. This old favourite can be enjoyed by the visually impaired child. Initially a one-to-one practice game with an adult may be necessary. The leader calls out what he is doing and the others follow his actions. When the visually impaired child is the leader, he may need some suggestions of what to do, as the possibilities are not as obvious to him.

Follow-the-Leader can also be played over an obstacle course, such as under a chair, over a stool, through a tunnel made out of a large box, in between cushions, under the table.

This game can be played with a very young child as a simple one-to-one game of imitation. Encourage the child to imitate your actions, movements, or sounds. Also imitate the child's actions, movements, and sounds. Blind children will need verbal descriptions.

Scavenger Hunt

Children are usually paired and given a list of items to find in their environment. When they have all the items, they bring them back to the adult. A time limit is set. The winning pair has the most correct items. This can be adapted for a younger visually impaired child, and can be played indoors or outdoors. The adult asks for one item. The child searches for it and takes it to the adult. The adult then asks for another item. What the objects are and how many are requested will depend on the child's interest and ability. At the end of the game, the adult guesses where the items were found and player and adult share the responsibility of replacing them. The adult can ask the child to pick out the items from a particular room and put only those away. This game helps a child learn the specific location of items in the home. When the child is proficient at this game, a kitchen timer can be used to provide competition. If a sighted child is also included in the game, the children can be paired or each can search for different items.

Bowling

Use plastic bleach bottles or tin cans for pins, and add coloured or regular tin foil for visual interest. Put a variety of things inside to provide different sounds, such as stones, rice, or macaroni. Place the pins by a wall, which will create a boundary so the ball will not go too far. The visually impaired child feels or sees where the pins are. Let him take two or three steps backwards and then roll a ball to knock the pins over. A variation is to lay a large metal garbage can on its side and roll or throw a ball into it.

Beanbag Throw

Put a broom handle across two chairs in front of a wall. On the handle hang one plastic bleach bottle with macaroni inside, or hang several close together to make it simpler for the blind child. Let the child feel the bottles, step back, and throw a beanbag to hit the bottles and make them rattle. To encourage use of vision, cover bottles with tin foil or paint them in bright colours. You could make your own beanbag with an odd sock filled with macaroni or dried beans.

Make a Splash

Put a bucket of water by the wall and let the child feel the bucket. Then have the child step back and throw a ball into the bucket and listen for the splash. He can then be encouraged to reach into the water and take out the ball.

This game, as well as bowling and the beanbag throw, could be played with other children. Where any child stands in relation to the bucket or bottle will depend on age and skill levels. Adjust the distance accordingly.

Easter Egg Hunt

For the visually impaired child an Easter Egg Hunt can be organized by using ribbon, tape, wool, or string (a different texture for each child). Each child finds several eggs along his route. The first egg could be hidden under a chair. Tie the ribbon from the chair to the next hiding place and so on until the ribbon has led a trail to all of the eggs. The child has to follow his ribbon to find all the Easter eggs. The more mature child may have to follow his trail under or over furniture, or under, over, or parallel to another child's trail.

Fun Quizzes or Car Games

These games can be played with an individual child at any quiet moment, in the doctor's waiting-room, or in the car. If more than one child plays, establish some simple rules. These are intended to be fun. They are not tests.

• Ask the child to think of all the things that would be needed to do an activity: swimming, riding, skating, washing the dishes, taking a bath, etc.
• Ask the child to think of a boy's name, a girl's name, the name of a man in his family, the name of a woman in his family, a dog's name, his teacher's name, etc.
• Ask the child questions related to the use of clothing. Would boots be worn in a living-room? Would a hat be worn in the shower? (Don't forget you may wear a shower cap in the shower.) Would a bathing-suit be worn outside on a snowy day?
• Ask the child how many things he can remember in the bathroom, toy-box, etc.
• In the car ask the child questions about the journey. Did the car turn right or left? Why did the car stop? What vehicle (bus, truck, motorcycle) passed the car? Is the car going fast or slow?
• Play the old familiar game of 'I went shopping and I bought.' For example, the first person begins by saying, 'I went shopping and I bought an orange.' The second person continues, 'I went shopping and I bought an orange and a piano.' Then the third person says, 'I went shopping and I bought an orange, a piano, and a rabbit,' and so on. The first one who forgets an item on the list is out. The last person left is the winner. The items in your list can be random or from a specific store; they can be small items, items bigger than the child, things that make a noise, things to eat, things to wear, etc.
• This is a car game, but can be used on other occasions too. The children can wear necklaces made of peanuts, which the older or sighted children have helped to make prior to the car trip. Everybody sings the song, 'Found a peanut, found a peanut.' Every time they come to the end of the verse, one peanut can be cracked open and eaten. To prevent a messy car and add to the enjoyment, each child could have a small container to put the shells in. When the lid is put on the container they will have a handmade maraca.

Table Games

Odd one out. On a table place two pieces of clothing or items needed for a specific activity. Add a third item that does not belong to the set. Ask the child to find the two appropriate items for the activity or, conversely, to find the item that does not belong. You can use items that are soft, or made of paper or wood, or have a pleasant smell, etc.

Concentration. At the preschool level, this is a game for two or three players. You need a set of cards with matching pairs. Most commercial card games for children contain matching cards. Your visually impaired child may be able to play with these. If the pictures on the cards are too busy, too small, unclear, or the contrast is not good, you will need to make your own. You could use an old set of playing-cards or cardboard from a box, the back of a writing-pad, or an old record sleeve.

If you make your own cards, they should be the same size and all cards should be identical on the back. The number of cards and what you put on the face side depend on the developmental level of your child or children. If using old playing-cards, the face side needs to be totally covered in plain paper first so the original picture does not show through and confuse the child. Stick on coloured construction paper to cover the face side. Be sure it does not overlap the sides. Paste on simple geometric shapes. Use black on white or another good colour contrast. Draw outlines with felt pen or colour in a solid shape.

For the totally blind child, outlined shapes can be made with string stuck onto the card, or for solid shapes you can use glue sprinkled with sand or salt. You can also use finger-paint instead of glue. Shapes can be made out of sandpaper, corrugated paper, or felt and stuck onto the card. For the more advanced child, cut a piece of construction paper the size of the card and mark out the desired shape on this with a series of pinpricks. Stick the construction paper onto the card, making sure the raised pinpricks are up.

Cards are placed face down on the table in two rows. It is a good idea to use a tray at first to provide a boundary. The first player turns up two cards and everybody calls out what they are. If the cards match, the player keeps them and has another turn. If they do not match, he turns them over, leaving them in the same place and giving other players time to visually or tactually identify the positions. Then it is the next player's turn, and so on, until all the cards are picked up. The player with the most cards is the winner. This can start as a simple matching game with only one or two shapes or

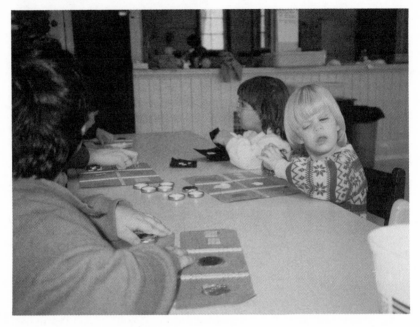

Playing textured bingo.

colours. This can be a car game if played on a baking sheet or metal tray with small pieces of magnetic tape on each card.

Dominoes. A simple matching game of dominoes can be played by using geometric shapes, coloured letters, or numbers. Dominoes can be made from an old set of dominoes or from strong cardboard, following suggestions given in the directions for Concentration.

Tic-tac-toe. This game is suitable for visually impaired, mature pre-schoolers. It can be played among themselves or with their sighted friends. Each of two players in turn places his piece on the board. The object of the game is to form your own pieces in a line of three horizontally, vertically, or diagonally, while preventing your opponent from doing the same. Some children are ready for a more challenging version, once they are familiar with the game. Each child can place an X or an O on the board only if he can answer a simple question correctly. Questions may be asked by a third child or adult, or the players may ask each other.

To make the board, cut a square of cardboard or wood to the

desired size. Divide into nine equal squares. Glue string on the cardboard to make the divisions. On wood, cut grooves or make ridges to make divisions. Each player will need five identical items that are different from his opponent's set, such as bottle tops or buttons.

Bingo or textured lotto. Simple bingo bases, approximately 10 inches by 10 inches (25.5 cm by 25.5 cm), can be made out of cardboard and divided into any number of squares you choose. To make divisions, stick on string or make outlines with white glue that will dry into raised ridges, or mark clearly with felt pen. For the playing pieces, cut out squares of cardboard the size of the squares on the bingo base. For partially sighted children, draw or cut and paste geometric shapes or simple pictures on the playing-cards and corresponding shapes or pictures on the base. For blind children, use simple items, such as buttons, paper-clips, bottle caps, or cover squares with different textures. Simple geometric shapes can also be used. At preschool level textured pictures are usually not understood by the congenitally blind child. This game can be played individually. The bingo base is given to the child and he is encouraged to examine each square. Remove the base while the child examines individual cards. After this he is ready to play.

Simple matching game. Place the individual cards on a small tray, box, or lid to provide a boundary. How many cards you use and whether you place them face up or down, in lines or at random, depends on the child's level of skill. The adult calls out the names on the cards one at a time and asks the child to find the corresponding square on the bingo base. When the child is competent he can play at matching the cards alone, racing the kitchen timer for excitement.

For a group game, you will need as many bingo bases as players. The leader has all the individual cards, picks one at a time at random and names the card. Each child covers the appropriate square on his base. Any items can be used to cover, such as poker chips, squares of paper, wrapped candy, or coins. (Using money gives the child the opportunity to become familiar with different coins.) The winner is the first child to have a full card.

CRAFTS

You can find good craft books in any library. Many of the ideas they

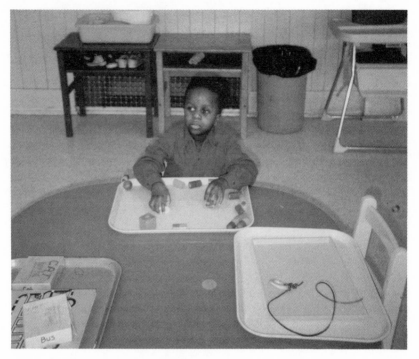

Blind children need clearly defined boundaries for their activities.

present can easily be used for partially sighted children. A few adaptations may be needed. Finding crafts that are meaningful for blind children is more difficult. The following crafts are suggested with the blind child in mind, but may be enjoyed by any child. Careful attention to detail is necessary when introducing crafts to visually impaired children. Here are some helpful hints when organizing crafts:

- Use muffin tins to separate items you are going to use.
- Baking sheets or trays provide boundaries.
- Garbage bags can be used as aprons.
- Have a ready-made item for the child to examine, so that he knows what he is making. Whenever possible, have examples of the item in different stages for the child to examine.
- Glue sticks are easy to use.
- When using glue or finger-paint, have a damp sponge or cloth available.
- Keep Scotch tape in its dispenser and show the child how to use it.

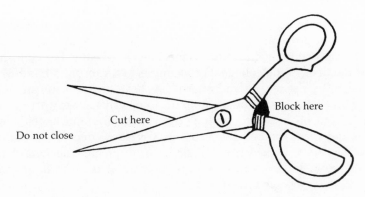

Blocking prevents scissor blades from closing completely,
making them easier to handle for the visually impaired child.

- If the child has difficulty using scissors, make a block using a wad of paper or cotton batting and tape in place between the handles, close to the pivot of the scissors. This prevents the scissor blades from completely closing. It is the complete closing and opening of the blades that usually give the blind child difficulty. Once the child has learned to control the scissors, the blocking will not be necessary. Use small scissors that are sharp enough to cut the material being used. Blunt scissors are frustrating.
- It is useful to have a stapler handy for securing material that the child has glued.
- For decorating craft items, save coloured foil candy wrappers or foil wrapping paper. Some hardware and building suppliers also carry foil tape.
- Display the child's work low enough so the child can explore it. He may need to be reminded that it is there.

Collages

Collages can be made from almost any small items and are limited only by your imagination. They can be used as pictures in a child's room or even as a frieze around a wall. They can be fun for the blind child, but also give him an opportunity to explore items he might not come in contact with at another time. Remember to call all items by their correct names and, depending on the maturity of the child, give a simple explanation of what the items are used for or where they are found. For example, nuts and bolts are used in the workshop; macaroni and rice are used for cooking; pine-cones grow on trees.

When possible, make some connections soon after the child has used the item in the collage. For example, you can put a handful of macaroni in a saucepan and after it has been boiled, you can show the child that it has become soft and can be eaten. Hardware can be pointed out on furniture, such as drawer handles and knobs. Pine-cones and sticks can be related to fires, Christmas decorations, or the trees they were picked from. Collages have greater meaning if the pieces are collected with an enthusiastic adult on a walk or from around the house. A few ideas for collages:

- *Nature:* cones, stones, twigs, leaves, sand, nuts, seeds, gravel, petals, stalks, thistles, shells, coral
- *Food items:* eggshells, dried beans, macaroni, rice, sugar, salt, orange or lemon peel, date pits, orange pips
- *Workshop:* nuts, bolts, nails, screws, washers (rubber and metal), hooks, pieces of chain, wood pieces or shavings, hinges, knobs, handles
- *Small containers:* pill bottles, tiny boxes, tins (no sharp edges), matchboxes, plastic boxes
- *Sewing notions:* spools, darning wool, dome fasteners, eyelets, buttons, hooks, pieces of tape, lace, rickrack braid, elastic, safety-pins
- *First-aid items:* cotton batting, Band-Aids, toothpicks, Q-Tips, pieces of gauze bandage
- *Desk oddments:* paper-clips (various sizes), pieces of eraser, small pencils, chalk, crayon, wax crayon or pencil shavings, elastic bands, old pens
- *Paper:* facial tissue, toilet tissue, cellophane, newspaper, brown paper, crepe paper, magazines, writing-paper, envelopes, stamps, tin foil, corrugated cardboard, wax paper, paper cups
- *Fabric:* velvet, corduroy, burlap, cotton, wool, felt, satin, silk, fake fur, carpet scraps, onion bags, nylon pantihose
- *Lids:* bottle tops, toothpaste tops, jar lids, corks
- *Tags and string:* pieces of string, rope, thread, garbage ties, bread tags, pipe-cleaners
- *Plastic and styrofoam:* pieces of plastic bags, garbage bags, freezer bags, styrofoam chips, meat and fruit trays, styrofoam cups
- *Jewellery:* all kinds of broken jewellery (single beads, brooches, strings of beads, chains, earrings, etc.)

There are many ways to make collages. The background can be newspaper, opened brown paper bags, cardboard, pieces of wood, an old tray or baking sheet, paper plates, etc. Paper must be secured firmly to a table or tacked to a bulletin-board. A bulletin-board also works well to secure paper or tin-foil plates.

Simple paste can be made from flour and water mixed together. This is good for paper or lightweight items, is inexpensive, and is easy for small children to use with fingers, popsicle sticks, or spoons for easy clean-up. Stick double-sided carpet tape to the background, so the child can place objects on it. Use one strip at a time, attaching a new strip as the one above is filled. Glue sticks are easy to handle and good for many items. White glue can be squeezed from a bottle or placed in a container and used like paste.

For very small children, flour-and-water paste spread over the bottom of a paper plate works well. The child places items on the paper plate at random. For a greater learning experience, older children can choose items from one category and paste at random or in patterns, or the child can use a variety of items. You can also divide the background by sticking on wool or string at corners, in strips or circles, and suggest that the child put specific items in certain areas: for example, macaroni in corner areas, rice in the centre square, and so on. This helps the child to understand patterns and then form his own.

Brown paper bags opened and taped together make good wall friezes. The friezes are best spread out on an uncarpeted floor or patio. Several children can work together, or if left in an out-of-the-way place, the child can add to it over a period of days or weeks. At kindergarten level, the child can make patterns using one type of item, such as tiny paper-clips around the edge of a paper plate, working in rows to a jumbo clip in the centre. Buttons or lids can also be used in this way. At this level, the child can also make small collages cut from a notice-board or ceiling tile and covered by sticking map pins in it. In a safe way, the child learns the meaning of 'sharp.'

Plaster of Paris collages. Plaster of Paris is inexpensive and obtainable from a hardware store. This is a variation of the paper collage. Mix plaster of Paris and water to form a smooth paste (pancake batter consistency). Pour into a container – paper plate, box, etc. Allow one or two minutes to set, then the child can put in the pieces. Plaster of Paris dries *very* fast so make small plaques that the child can cover quickly before the plaster has set. Plaster can be left in paper or tin-foil plates and small boxes, or removed to make wall plaques. Remember to insert a small hanger before the plaster dries. A garbage bag tie works well. If using boxes that will be removed later, line with foil or waxed paper or the plaster will stick to the boxes and be difficult to remove.

Collage jewellery. Cut small circles, squares, triangles, or irregular shapes of cardboard. Punch a hole in the top of each shape. Use tiny items such as seeds, rice, sand, shells, beads, and beans to cover the cardboard in patterns. Thread yarn or cord through the hole to form a pendant. To make the pendant lie flat, fold yarn in half before threading. Push loop at fold through the hole and then push the ends of the cord through this loop and pull tight. For a brooch, tape a safety-pin to the back of the shape slightly above centre. For a buckle, cut the cardboard a little larger than for a brooch or pendant and punch two holes on each side. For a belt, thread ribbon or wool through the holes and tie at the back of the waist.

Christmas Wreath

Cut out a cardboard circle about the size of a dinner plate. Cut out a smaller circle in the centre to form a wreath. Punch one hole at the outside edge of the cardboard circle. Have the child thread a pipe-cleaner or string through the hole for a hanger. The child can cover the wreath with pine-cones, nuts, Christmas decorations, pine needles, cinnamon sticks, and felt pieces. Dip the articles into a saucer of white glue. Cones can be plain, painted, sprayed, or covered with sparkles. The cardboard base can first be covered with felt. If the child is partially sighted, the base can be painted. Another option is to wind ribbon around a painted or felt-covered base and staple or stick in place. The child fills in spaces between the ribbon with a choice of materials.

Decorating Small Tins or Boxes

It may be helpful for some children, who have difficulty using their hands, to fill the tin with heavy stones, etc. Cardboard boxes can be pinned firmly to a bulletin-board on a table. By securing the box or tin, you give the blind child freedom to use both hands for finding and sticking on items. It can also be helpful to place the weighted tin on a lazy Susan.

Dish Gardens

Some blind children will enjoy these; for others they will have little meaning. Dish gardens are still the basic collage idea. For the base, use a tin-foil plate or tray. Use soil or sand slightly dampened, or even plaster of Paris. Items can be collected on a nature walk. Make small flower-beds with tiny flowers, using small pieces of evergreen or shrubs for trees. You can make a pool or lake, using a small sardine or tuna tin and twigs to form a bridge. Gravel and small stones make paths.

For this craft to be meaningful, the child must have a well-developed concept of a garden. However, a younger child can make just a garden path out of gravel or flat stones and then walk his fingers along the path, but only after he has walked along a small garden path, so that he can make a comparison.

Wind Chimes Mobile

You will need two metal coat-hangers, old keys or metal items that can be threaded on the hangers (nuts, washers, etc.), wire garbage ties and electric duct or plastic tape or wire. An adult prepares the mobiles by using electric duct or plastic tape to fasten hangers together at right angles, taping where they meet in the centre. Twist or cut off one hook and tape the cut end and remaining hook firmly together. Show the child how to push wire ties through holes in the keys and bend and twist them tightly together. Thread all the items before hanging them on the hanger.

Twisting threaded items onto the hanger may require a slightly different movement from any the child knows. If you have a ready-made wind chime, the child should have explored it first so he will have some understanding of what he is doing. If not, the adult can thread two keys onto the hanger. Show the child and let him hear their sound. Next, show the child how to bend the tie over the hanger and again twist the tie tightly. The child continues adding keys or other metal items to the hanger. When keys are in place, the child can be shown how to hold the hanger hook and gently shake or rotate it back and forth and listen to the pleasing sound. The mobile can be hung where there is a breeze.

You may need to tighten the wire ties after small children have bent them; however, let them try first. Blind children, if shown very precisely how to do it, will usually manage all on their own. The activity is good to strengthen little fingers. You can prevent all the keys from bunching up together by sticking a little tape between a few keys to keep them spread out more evenly; however, some sliding is desirable.

Windmill

You will need a square of paper – construction paper is colourful and easy to work with. Use any size, but small windmills about 3 to 4 inches (7.5 to 10 cm) in diameter are easier for young children to make. A hatpin, stick or long pencil with an eraser on the end, stapler, and glue stick or Scotch tape are also needed. It is helpful to have several partially made windmills so the child can explore different stages of the process before attempting each step independently. To begin with, the adult folds the paper diagonally and allows the child to help press it down to crease. Open up the paper again and let the child refold it. The child at kindergarten level should be shown how the corners match on the section just folded and then repeat the whole process independently, matching the opposite corners. Encourage the child to examine the creases and find the centre where the two lines cross. Examine both sides of the paper. The child should be given a paper to practise cutting if not already familiar with using scissors.

Using a stapler, the adult then puts a line of staples on the right side (if child is left-handed, on the left side) of each crease to approximately a finger-width from the centre point. This will be the child's guide for cutting. Show the child how to feel the line of staples and where they end. The child holds scissors close to fingers and cuts slowly along the staples, using fingers to guide the cutting. Small windmills are easier to make, as the child can hold the paper and feel the staples on both sides as he cuts. Blind children at kindergarten level, and even some at nursery school level, can often do this very well – sometimes better than the children who have vision!

Now show the child how to bend the alternate unstapled sides to the centre point. Remind the child that this time he does not crease it; show the model. Using glue sticks or small pieces of tape, attach each point to the centre. If using tape, let the child practise detaching small pieces of tape from the dispenser first. When all corners are secured at the centre and *glue is dry*, stick the hatpin through the centre. An older child can do this himself. If glue is not dry, the pin

Bend alternate cut corners to the centre

Staple ridge/cut line

Hatpin at centre secures
the four cut corners

An easy-to-make windmill is attached to a stick or pencil.

will become sticky as it is pushed through and the windmill will not
spin as freely. If this happens, pull the pin out and clean it. Stick the
pin into the pencil eraser and the windmill is complete. Show the
child how to blow and listen to it spin. Blind children who cannot
see any movement can be shown how to hold a hand close to the
spinning edges so the windmill blade just touches and makes a
clicking noise as it spins. For children with light perception or very
limited vision, attaching sticky coloured tin-foil tape to the tips of the
windmill blades adds interest. Use windmills outside or place them
where there is a breeze – e.g., near windows or heat registers.

Greeting Cards

Here are some ideas for cards that would be meaningful for a blind child to give or receive. Old cards can be used. Stick on plain paper to cover the original picture. Construction paper, lightweight card stock, or regular paper can also be used.

Birthday cards

- *Candle card:* Stick a birthday cake candle onto a card or stick several candles, according to the birthday child's age. A small bow can be added at the base of the candle. To ensure the child understands the significance of the candle, place a small piece of tin foil on a muffin and stick a candle into the centre. Light the candle and let the blind child experience warmth and melted wax as the candle burns down. The child blows out the candle and compares the size of the burned-down candle to that of an unused candle. Never take concept development for granted.
- *Candy card:* Cut a shape (square, circle, triangle) out of felt or card. The child sticks this outline onto the centre of a card. He then sticks wrapped candies onto the shape. Explain to the blind child that it is a nice card to feel and is also a tasty gift. You could limit the number of candies to the birthday child's age, or glue on seven candies and explain to the child that he has put enough candies on the card so his friend can have one candy each day for a whole week. (Of course the recipient may choose to eat them all at once. Let the blind child know this could happen!)
- To make a *surprise pocket card*, you can use a pocket cut from an old garment or make one out of felt or heavy fabric that does not fray too easily. To prevent fraying, put glue on the edges. The child sticks the ready-made pocket onto the centre of the card. Decorate the card as desired with lace, buttons, bows, etc. The surprise inside the pocket could be a wrapped candy, a cookie wrapped in tin foil, a small ring, a musical box or squeaker used for putting in home-made stuffed toys, a brooch, a small fragrant guest soap, etc.
- To make a *fragrant card*, purchase or make a tiny lavender bag ahead of time. To make, use lightweight fabric and cut two circles about 3 inches (7.5 cm) in diameter. The child glues the circle edges together, leaving a small opening. When the glue is dry, the child puts lavender into the bag using a small kitchen funnel or paper funnel. Alternatively, use pomander spices or cotton batting sprinkled with perfume; however, the smell will not last long and the adult may need to add more perfume before the card is given. When fragrance has been added, the child glues the opening closed

and sticks the fragrant bag onto the card. Little bows can be added for additional decoration if desired.

Christmas cards
- Make tiny wreaths, as described under Collages, and stick these onto the card.
- Stick candy cane and bow onto the card.
- As suggested for fragrant birthday cards, but use spice instead of perfume, cinnamon, cloves, etc., and decorate with bows and small nuts in shells. (You might like to boil a few cloves and cinnamon sticks to allow the child to experience a Christmassy fragrance.)
- Make a small paper chain and place on the card.
- Stick on a card a small twig cut from a fir tree. Add tiny Christmas decorations or make balls from tin foil.
- Thread a few tiny bells and glue to the card. Stick bows above the threads.
- A more elaborate Christmas card can be made by using a pantihose card or heavy paper. Fold to form a greeting card. Cut a door in the centre of the card front. The child can make and stick a tiny wreath on the door. Glue a paper chain or a fir twig to the inside of the card. Explain to the blind child how the door opens to reveal the Christmas decorations.

Easter cards
- Make a cross from small twigs or use popsicle sticks. (Cut popsicle sticks for short sides.) The child sticks pieces in place and glues ribbon, rickrack, or lace around the edge of the card. Explain the significance of the card.
- Decorate with broken eggshells. Explain the significance.
- Model an Easter-egg shape out of play dough or tin foil. Add ribbon and stick to the card. Use a hard-boiled egg as a model for shape.

Valentine cards
- Cut a heart shape out of red felt or lightweight card stock and glue to the card.
- Prick the shape of a heart from the back of the card using a pin. Turn the card over. The child feels the outline and applies glue within the pricked area. Sprinkle salt and sugar on the glued area of the card.
- Using a mesh board, the child traces his own hand and fills in the

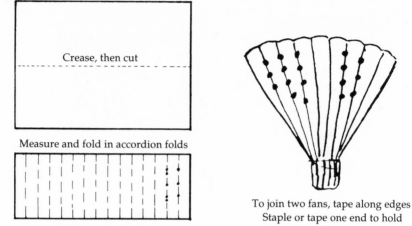

Crease, then cut

Measure and fold in accordion folds

To join two fans, tape along edges
Staple or tape one end to hold

Paper fans are simple to make and can be decorated as desired.

outline by using wax crayons while the paper is still on the mesh board. The child will be able to feel the area he has filled in.

All cards have the child's name and message written in braille, print, or both. Sandwich bags make good envelopes.

Christmas and Party Chains

Using pinking shears, cut strips of construction paper 1 inch (2.5 cm) wide. The child can practise cutting along any folded line and cut a few strips himself. Use a tray to provide a boundary. Put the strips in a low-sided cake pan and place the pan on the left side of the tray. Put a glue stick and scissors in a container on the right side. It is important for a blind child to have organized space. In this case it will prevent paper strips from getting accidentally glued. Sticky strips will be very frustrating for the blind child. Place a damp sponge and towel above the tray in front of the child.

The child takes a strip and glues both ends, forming the first link in the chain. He takes another strip and threads it through the first link and sticks the ends together. Encourage the child to count the loops of the growing paper chain periodically. Compare with siblings or other children who may be making a chain at the same time. Making a chain can also help the blind child's understanding of space. Choose an area such as the headboard on his bed, a door, a picture, or a bookshelf. Encourage the child to take his chain to see how much longer it must be to reach across an area. A picture can be taken down and placed beside the child so he can measure against it as he makes the chain. If the chain is to be hung high, allow the child to climb onto a chair or stepladder to put up his decoration. If the child has light perception, use tin foil in the chain.

Weaving

For preschool children use heavy cardboard or wood as a base and hat elastic (round) as the vertical thread. Weave with wool, strips of cloth, etc. Elastic makes it easier for the child to manipulate over-and-under movement.

Fans

Fans are good to make on a hot day or to use as party or Christmas decorations. You will need paper, a stapler or Scotch tape, and glue. A single-hole punch, coloured wool, and tissue or cellophane paper are optional.

Take a sheet of construction paper or any heavy writing-paper. If using typewriter-size paper, fold and cut the sheet in half lengthwise. You will now have two strips approximately $4\frac{1}{4}$ inches by 11 inches (11 cm by 28 cm). Draw vertical lines approximately $\frac{1}{2}$ inch (1 cm) apart crosswise along the strips. If working with a partially sighted child, draw lines with a black felt-tip pen on light-coloured paper. If a ruler is not handy, fold the strip of paper in half, short sides together, and continue folding in this manner until you have a wad of paper $\frac{1}{2}$ inch (1 cm) thick. Open it up and flatten it out. You will now have creases evenly spaced. Fold the paper again, this time in accordion folds. Use your lines as a guide. Crease firmly then open out. Do this with both strips.

Now show the child how to fold the paper to make a fan. Fold the first flap up and then turn the paper over and show the child how to fold away from himself (use the body as a reference point) each time he turns the paper. The previously creased paper will make it easier to fold. As the wad gets bigger, the child will begin to understand what he is doing. When it is all folded, staple or tape one end together. Kindergarten children will be able to do this themselves. Now the child can open up the fan. Encourage the child to repeat with the second piece; help only if necessary. When the two small fans are made, show the child how to glue them together to make one big fan. Staple or tape the ends together.

An option is to punch a hole at or along each crease, which gives a pretty effect. Show the child the confetti he has made from the hole-punching and explain that confetti is used at weddings. The older or more dextrous child can punch one or more rows of holes on each crease and thread wool or narrow lace through the holes to decorate the fan. Cut and glue the ends in place. Be sure the fan is stretched wide open before cutting the wool or lace and gluing the ends.

Partially sighted children or older siblings may like to punch holes before fastening the ends of the fan and stick tissue or cellophane paper behind the holes. This gives a pretty stained glass effect. Punch two or three holes so they overlap and make a bigger, longer hole.

Simple Maracas

You will need plastic bottles and sticks about 8 or 12 inches (20.5 cm or 30.5 cm) long, depending on the length of the bottle. Paint stirrers work well for wide-mouth bottles. For narrow-mouth bottles, use bamboo plant supports or find sticks on a nature walk. You will also need Scotch tape in a dispenser and some beans, stones, rice, or small buttons for sound. Stick-on Christmas pom-poms or bows and ribbon are optional decorations.

Place a few of the chosen sound-makers into the bottle, then insert the stick in the bottle. Show the child how to detach small pieces of tape from the dispenser and attach the stick to the bottle by covering the hole. He continues to add tape until the stick is firmly in place and his fingers cannot feel any gaps around the mouth of the bottle. To decorate, cut a piece of ribbon and place it around the neck of the bottle, tying it firmly in place and leaving the ends hanging. (Bells could be attached to ends.) Stick on a pom-pom or some foil paper. If the child is partially sighted, the maraca can also be painted. The child can shake his maraca by holding the handle. Encourage the child to make two or three maracas and compare different sounds, or make them with friends, each child using a different sound-maker. If the children save a little of the sound-makers that they have placed into the bottles, they can each compare the left-over sound-makers with the different sounds of the maracas. Use the maracas in an action song, such as 'Mrs Murphy Had a Band' in Chapter 6.

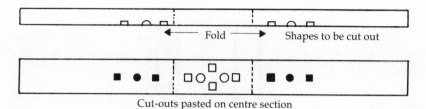

Fold →   Shapes to be cut out

Cut-outs pasted on centre section

A felt belt can be decorated with cut-out shapes.

Maracas can be hung in the child's room, perhaps on the door. For very small children, have the child put a few sound-makers in a bottle; encourage him to screw on the lid.

Making a Belt out of Felt

Cut a 2-inch (5-cm) strip of felt to fit halfway around the child's waist. Fold the strip in half lengthwise. You will now have a 1-inch (2.5-cm) strip. Press to make a sharp crease. Find the centre by folding the strip in half end to end, mark with a pin, then measure 2 inches (5 cm) on either side of the centre pin and mark these points with pins. Remove the centre pin. This 4-inch (10-cm) centre area will not be cut. Show the child the belt and crease and explain that he is going to cut out shapes on the crease on each side of the centre. To help the child, you can precut shapes out of card and pin to the belt. Suggested shapes: two triangles and half a circle. On one side of the belt's centre, place the bases of the triangles and half circle against the crease, with the circle between the triangles. Pin in place. The child can cut around the card. When the belt is unfolded, there will be cut-out diamonds with a circle in the centre. Partially sighted children may like to paste contrasting coloured felt behind the cut-out spaces. The child glues cut-out shapes onto the centre section. He can feel the raised areas. Other small items, such as small buttons, can also be glued on. To finish the belt, an adult stitches elastic to tie around the waist or stitches tape to each end of the belt.

Headband

Sew elastic to a strip of felt. To make headband, glue on shapes, sparkles, or small buttons. A tiny bell also adds interest.

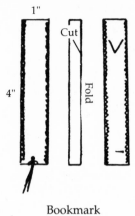

Bookmark

Felt or Paper Bookmark

Cut a 1-inch by 4-inch (2.5-cm by 10-cm) strip of paper or felt. Fold
in half lengthwise and pin if using felt. About 1½ inches (4 cm) from
the top, make a 1-inch (2.5-cm) diagonal cut from the centre crease.
When bookmark is opened there will be a V-shape that will slip over
a page. Alternatively, punch a hole at the centre bottom and thread
a small piece of ribbon. Decorate with narrow rickrack down each
side of the bookmark.

Bookmark from an Old Envelope

Use a corner of a used envelope. Measure 2 inches (5 cm) along each
side from the corner and cut diagonally. The bookmark will slip over
a corner of a page. The child puts glue on the bookmark and
sprinkles on sparkles.

Doorstop

The child fills a plastic bottle with sand and screws on the lid tightly.
Decorate with felt, paper, tin foil, etc. in collage style.

Paper Hat

To make a paper hat, take a *folded* newspaper. Place on table, open
side closest to self. Fold layers of paper in half crosswise. Crease and

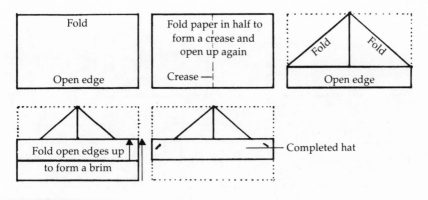

Paper hats.

open. Fold top corners to line up with centre crease. You now have a point looking like a sail or a tepee. Separate unfolded paper at bottom and fold up one layer at the front and the back. This will form the hat brim. Staple the brim together above the crown. The child can now decorate with paper, cotton batting, ribbons, etc., using glue or safety-pins.

Hand and Foot Moulds

Make plaster of Paris moulds of hands or feet – the child's and an adult's – to compare sizes. Into paper plates or tin-foil plates pour plaster of Paris, which has been mixed to a smooth paste with water, about the consistency of fairly thick pancake mix (colour the water if a tint is desired). When the plaster is just beginning to dry, the child presses his hand or foot into it. A picture hanger can be attached if a plaque is desired. Partially sighted children can paint the background or the indented print. Blind children can sprinkle on sand or sparkles while the plaster is still wet, or use glue to attach the sparkles when the plaster is totally dry.

Baskets

This is an easy craft that is quick and simple; and the product *can be used by the child.* The baskets can be filled with many different items, such as beads, blocks, small toys, mitts, socks, jewellery, cassette tapes. The child can also make and fill them with cookies, candies, fruit, or nuts to give as gifts at Christmas, birthdays, etc. The baskets

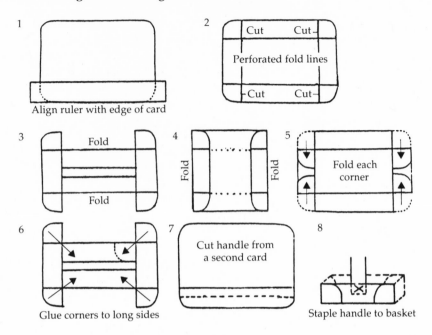

Baskets make useful gifts and storage containers.

can sit side by side on a shelf or in a drawer and are easy to carry, and help the child organize his own belongings. Most important, even a young blind child can learn to make them. If time is limited, the foil and cards can be precut and the child just does the gluing.

You will need two white cards, similar to those found in pantihose packages, approximately 6 inches by 9 inches (15 cm by 23 cm), ruler, pencil (or black felt pen if child is partially sighted), scissors, glue stick (or any glue with a stick for easy spreading), six paper-clips, and a stapler. If the child has no vision, you will need a folded newspaper, a hat pin, or a dressmaker's wheel.

Line ruler up with edge of card and hold firmly in place. An easy way to do this is to place card and ruler a fraction over the edge of the table or thickly folded newspaper so the child can *feel* if the ruler and card are aligned. Draw a pencil line or perforate using the pin or dressmaker's wheel along the edge of the ruler. When the card is turned over, the blind child will be able to feel the perforated line. The perforated line also makes the card easier to bend. Repeat on the remaining three sides of the card. Show the child how the lines meet at the corners. Cut to the corner point on the long side as shown in diagram. Bend all sides to crease and open the long sides first, then the short ends of the card, and then each corner. Bend the short and long sides, then glue the corners to the long sides. Fasten with paper-clips until glue is dry. To make the handle, cut a strip from the second card. Glue the handle to the long sides of basket. Hold with a paper-clip or staple. If lining with foil or waxed paper for cookies or candies, place the lining in basket before gluing on the handle.

Play Dough

This play dough will stay soft indefinitely when stored in an airtight container. You will need:

2 cups	all-purpose flour	500 mL
1 tbsp	alum (available in drugstores)	15 mL
$\frac{1}{2}$ cup	salt	125 mL
$1\frac{1}{2}$ cups	water	375 mL
1 tbsp	vegetable oil	15 mL
few drops	food colouring if desired	few drops
few drops	peppermint, lemon, or orange for fragrance	few drops

In large bowl, mix together flour and alum. Set aside. In saucepan heat salt, water, and oil just to boiling. Pour into flour mixture. Let cool slightly, then knead until combined. (The child can help with the kneading.) Add food colouring and fragrance and knead some more. Store inside ziplock plastic bags or containers with plastic lids.

Finger-Paint

2 cups	flour	500 mL
$\frac{1}{4}$ cup	sugar	50 mL
1 tsp	powdered paint	5 mL
$\frac{1}{2}$ cup	salt	125 mL
$1\frac{1}{2}$ cups	water	375 mL

Mix together. Sugar and salt give the finger-paint texture.

Pomander

This is a simple craft that young visually impaired children can participate in. For it to be fully meaningful, there are certain conceptual prerequisites. Even if the following concepts are not understood, this craft can still be used to develop concepts, to practise fine-motor skills, and to provide sensory input.

- A visually impaired child should understand an orange as a whole fruit. Many small visually impaired children have not handled an orange, only orange juice or peeled segments of an orange.
- A visually impaired child should understand that clothes can be kept in drawers or hung in closets. Young visually impaired children frequently have no idea where clothes are stored or that they are laundered. Clothes are placed out for them or handed to them.
- Young visually impaired children need to be made aware of the many pleasant and unpleasant smells in their environment. They also need to know that smells and fragrances can be transferred to other nearby items (for example, cigarette smoke can permeate clothing and leave a residual odour).
- The idea of giving needs to be fostered. The very nature of visual impairment necessitates that things are done for the child. To counteract the attitude that the world revolves around him, find opportunities for the child to do things for others. Making gifts is just one way. Think through all the steps before beginning. Be aware of how much more carefully this needs to be done when working with a visually impaired child. Collect all the items needed for the activity, including a damp sponge or cloth and towel for wiping hands. Remember, for children who explore primarily by using their hands, it is important to have the opportunity to clean them as often as they feel they need to.

You will need a damp sponge or cloth and towel, a tray (a baking sheet works well), an apron (this can be made out of a garbage bag and masking tape), string or elastic, a knitting needle or skewer, scissors, a toilet roll, two medium-size oranges with firm skins, a handful of cloves in a dish, pipe-cleaners or chenille stems, ribbons for a small bow, a sharp knife. A finished pomander is helpful. It takes the place of a picture. The child can examine it to understand what he is going to make.

To make an apron, fold the garbage bag in half lengthwise. Cut off the top corner at folded edge to make a hole for the head (don't make it too large). Cut armholes in the sides (long enough to allow freedom of movement). You can use these aprons many times if you reinforce the neck and armholes with masking tape and cut the bag to the appropriate length. Tie around waist with string or use elastic. Be sure the apron fits comfortably, or the child may not focus on the activity.

Do not hurry. Talk to the child and encourage conversation. For non-verbal children use language and touch. Spark interest and have fun together. With younger children, the first six steps can be done one day and the pomander made the following day.

1 Place a tray in front of the child. Always give a boundary to a space. Place a damp sponge or cloth and towel on the table close to the child.

2 Place oranges on the tray.

3 Compare the size of the oranges to the size of the child's hand. (His body is the child's reference point.) Feel the texture and smell the orange before cutting.

4 The adult cuts the peel of one orange in four pieces, leaving them attached at the base. Partially separate segments of the orange by pushing your thumb in at the top. Let the child explore different parts of the orange, talk about the orange juice and/or segments the child had at breakfast. Place the cut orange in the child's palm and show him how to use his fingers to push the partially separated segments back to the orange's original shape. Place an uncut orange in the child's other hand for comparison.

5 Share an orange – taste and discuss. Squeeze it to make juice. Encourage the child to try picking up an orange pit with his fingers and try again using only his lips. Help him experience. You are not teaching table manners right now. Remind the child that a damp sponge or cloth is available for wiping his hands.

6 Wipe the tray clean and point out the difference between the sticky and clean tray.

7 Place one whole orange on the tray in front of the child and a dish with cloves on his dominant side. (Is your child left- or right-handed?) Tell him where the cloves are to reinforce the concept of right and left. Place a damp sponge or cloth beside him as before.

8 The child explores the cloves – discuss the smell, feel, and taste.

9 Feel and discuss the skewer to be used for punching holes. Punch a hole in the orange and let the child feel the hole. The child punches a hole and feels it.

10 Show the child how to keep his finger on the hole and reach for

a clove with the other hand. (Visually impaired children often need to be encouraged to use two hands.) Push a clove into the hole. Repeat this step until the orange is covered. If the child finds this tedious, the adult should take some turns at putting in the cloves. Explain that the cloves need to be about a finger-width apart because the orange will shrink as it dries. Show the child a completed pomander.

11 Feel the orange covered with cloves and discuss. Can the orange roll as well as it did before? Smell the spicy smell and talk about how it will make clothes closets or drawers smell nice.

12 The adult and child together push a knitting needle or screw-driver through the orange. Kindergarten children can usually do this alone. Even a blind child who is younger can do this successfully if he understands exactly what is required. You must help the child understand what it means to make a hole right through. Show how a knitting needle or skewer goes through an orange or put it through the centre of the toilet paper roll to demonstrate.

13 Encourage the child to play with the extra pipe-cleaner, feeling how soft it is, how it bends and retains its shape. Compare this with the ribbon. This concept can be understood visually by the sighted child, but needs to be taught to the blind child.

14 Explain to the child that the pipe-cleaner or chenille stem is going to be pushed through the hole in the orange made by the skewer. Help the child make a knot or bend one end of the pipe-cleaner or chenille stem, explaining that this will prevent the orange from falling off.

15 Remove the skewer, help the child push the free end of the pipe-cleaner or chenille stem through the hole in the orange.

16 Cut the pipe-cleaner, leaving an end long enough to make a loop at the top to hang. If preferred, thread a ribbon through for a bow.

17 Tie the ribbon into a bow for the child. If the child can manage it, he can tie the bow himself or help the adult.

18 The pomander is now complete. Place it in a warm, dry place, such as the top of the refrigerator or near an air register. Explain to the child that the pomander must be allowed to dry and get hard and shrink as discussed earlier, that the nice smell will stay for many months and give clothes and drawers a lovely fragrance, and that this would make a pleasing Christmas or birthday gift for a favourite person. It takes a week or so to dry. As

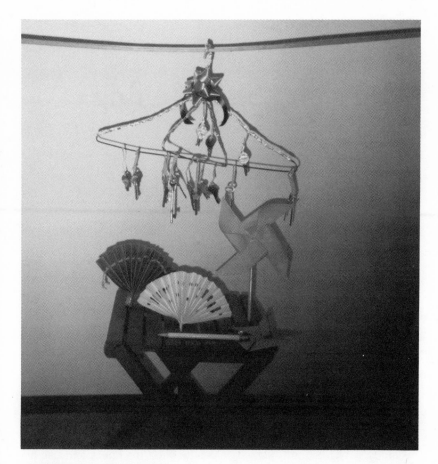

A selection of home-made toys.

the pomander dries, show the child each day how it becomes
harder and smaller as it shrinks.

19 Give the child opportunities to repeat the activity. With each
repetition his understanding will increase and he will be able to
participate more fully. Making pomanders for various family
members will give purpose to the activity.

EIGHT

Walks and Story-telling

A walk with a visually impaired child can be an enjoyable or a difficult experience. The following examples offer some suggestions that will help to give walks focus and meaning. We suggest four different types of walks. You can do them individually or combine some or all, depending on the time available. Whether you use these ideas or not, *the important thing is that you have fun together.*

Body Awareness Walk

Walk to improve body awareness and encourage freedom of movement. As you walk together, notice how your child moves his body. Is his head up? His back straight? Are his arms swinging loosely at his sides? Are his hand relaxed? Does he bend his knees and use his feet appropriately? When a child cannot observe how other people move, a walk provides a fun way to gain some of that information and increase his awareness of how his own body moves. If you notice some specific problem, you can include body movements that will help him overcome this difficulty.

Whether in an urban or rural area, your surroundings can provide a natural gymnasium. Your child might enjoy it if you chant or sing a favourite tune to give rhythm to body movements as you walk. Use your surroundings to create specific actions. For example, curbs, stairs, low walls, and slopes provide opportunities to step up, climb, or run up and down. Logs and boulders can be used for climbing or standing on to reach up to touch the leaves of a tree; park benches can be sat on or jumped off of; doors and gates open and close; trees provide low branches to climb and swing on, and there are cones, leaves, or fruit to be picked; fire hydrants, small posts, and poles are good for stretching arms around.

Talk about body movements in action. For example, 'I bent my knees when I stepped onto the curb'; 'Let's see if we can get up without bending our knees. It's difficult, isn't it?'; 'You'll have to stretch your arms up straight close to your head to reach this branch I am shaking'; 'I'm swinging my arms as I walk. Are you?'

Move in many different ways – walk, take big steps or small steps, run, jog, skip, hop, jump, lift feet high, crawl, roll, take side-steps, walk on heels, walk on toes, bend over a low branch or rail and find your toes. Whisper and shout in a tunnel to hear the echo. Blow dandelion seed heads. Run and jump until you are huffing and puffing, then take deep breaths and fill up your lungs. Sit down and rest.

To give an idea of distance and boundaries, suggest walking, running, etc., between two fire hydrants, from the front door to the garden gate, or across the driveway or path.

Exploration Walk

An exploration walk increases the child's knowledge of a small area of his environment and sparks his curiosity about the world in general. This is a short walk that takes a long time! Together you explore the immediate environment, perhaps a park, garden, school yard, parking lot, the block, your home, a school, church hall, part of a shopping plaza, or store. On this walk you explore details and build information that a sighted child can gain incidentally through vision. Take time together to search, examine, and discuss. As you do so, help your child become aware of many of the things that you may have previously taken for granted. You may not travel very far, but this walk will be as tiring for you as a long walk. It will be exciting for your child and rewarding for both of you. Here are some examples of detailed exploration.

Gate. Consider its construction – its hinges, latches, bolts, and gateposts. For partially sighted children, examine whether the gate is painted, and if so, what colour. How does it open and close, and what is its purpose? What is its size in relation to the child – big enough to admit a car or just a person? Is there a ledge to be climbed or swung on? What kind of a noise does the gate make when it is opened or closed – a squeak, a bang, or clunk? Sound can also indi-

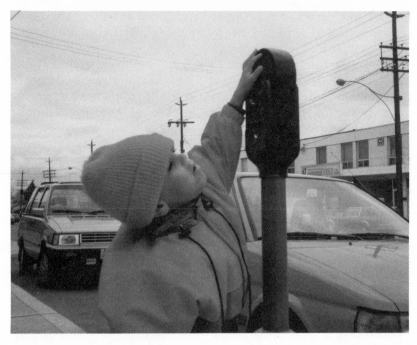

Finding the slot for the coins.

cate weight. Sounds can be confusing to the visually impaired child, so explain and discuss.

Rural mailbox. Explore its construction details carefully. Discuss who uses the mailbox. Is there a name on the box? A partially sighted child can be encouraged to find the name. Make the connection between the name on the mailbox and the person who lives in the nearby house. Explore the inside of the box, perhaps talk into the mailbox and hear the different sounds of your voices. As the child explores the box, you can point out a clue that would indicate a bird had perched there; perhaps there are bird droppings. Encourage the child to listen quietly to see if there are any birds around. At a later date, visit a pet store to learn more about birds.

Shoe store. Make friends with your local sales-people. Have fun exploring the store on a day that is not busy. This is a good opportunity for making comparisons – sizes, styles, and characteristics of shoes and purses. Examine running shoes, slippers, work boots,

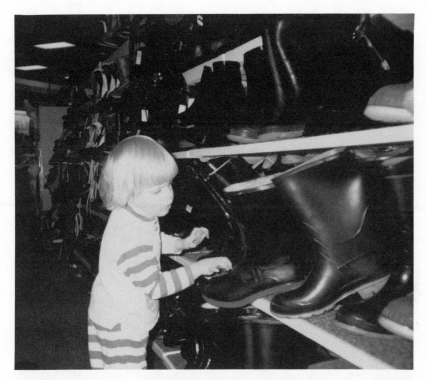

Who wears these boots? Specialty stores give good opportunities for comparisons.

snow-boots, ballet slippers, sandals, high-heel shoes, low-heel shoes, wedges, laces, Velcro, buttons, buckles, bows, zippers, bags, shoulder straps and hand straps, outside and inside pockets and flaps. What are they made of? Note the table, shelves, objects attached to walls and hung from the ceiling, the stacks of boxes. This visit, or several visits over a period of time, will provide information for interesting conversations, such as on travel, occupation, fashion, and coordinating colours. It is also an opportunity for the partially sighted child to identify colour, shades, and shapes.

In all your exploration walks notice the sounds, smells, textures under feet and hands, air temperature, weather conditions, etc. Exploration walks concentrate on small areas. The child needs to understand that these areas may be part of his walk to school or perhaps the store is one he passes regularly.

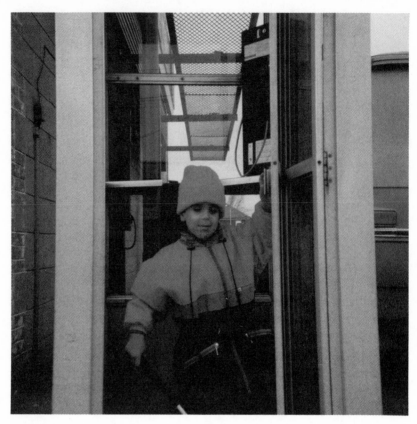

'Who answers this phone?'

Conversation Walk

This activity focuses on conversation and builds information about the purpose of the walk. On this walk, less attention is given to the environment. Conversation concentrates on why you are going to a destination and what you plan to do when you arrive. On your return trip, discuss what you did and highlight points of interest to tell other family members. Also discuss what you will do when you get home. Helping the child prepare for the walk will make it more meaningful. When talking with your child you limit his ability to converse if you only ask questions. Try to make interesting statements and build information onto his comments and responses.

Shopping to buy something for breakfast tomorrow. Conversation topics can include favourite breakfast foods; types of food eaten for breakfast; what will be purchased; the store you are going to; where the food is shelved; the kind of container it will be in; how to pay for it; how to carry it home; the people and things in the store.

A visit to the neighbour, Mrs Brown. Conversation topics can include the route to Mrs Brown's; whether she lives in a house or an apartment; whether she is on your side of the road or whether you have to cross the road. (Does your child know that the road has two sides and that there may be buildings on each side?) Conversation can also centre on Mrs Brown's family and pets. Are you taking anything for Mrs Brown? What will you do when you get there? Compare Mrs Brown's furniture with yours. How will Mrs Brown know you are at her door? How will you greet Mrs Brown? What does Mrs Brown like visitors to do with their shoes when they go into her house?

Going to the park. Conversation topics can include the playground equipment; favourite activities in the park; noises in the park; how hot the slide becomes in the sun; where to find a shady spot; listening for the bell of the ice-cream vendor; choosing an ice-cream; how quickly it may melt in the heat; friends you might meet. Recall the last visit to the park.

Sensory Walks

Sensory walks help the adult to become more tuned into and aware of the blind child's sensory experiences. Walk quietly together, just enjoying each other's company. Listen, feel, and be aware of your own and your child's reactions to the environment. Consciously tune into the sensory experiences around you. Make occasional brief comments to the child, such as about the rustle of the wind through the trees; how your clothes or hair blow in the breeze; the smell of a car exhaust or a fragrant bush; the buzz of a bee or insect; the sound of a lawnmower or a snowplough; the contrast of bright sunshine and shadow. Be aware of the feel of the child's hand in yours. Is he tense, excited, or relaxed? What non-verbal message is he giving you? Practising this walk on your own will enhance your understanding of the child.

THE ART OF STORY-TELLING

For many children, stories are a happy, daily event. However, young blind children and non-verbal and multihandicapped children are often not told stories. They too would enjoy and benefit from hearing them. In this chapter we will discuss some of the reasons why stories are often not told to visually impaired children, and offer suggestions on how to make them a useful teaching tool and an enjoyable experience for all children.

Barriers to Story-telling

Perhaps the most obvious reason why stories are not told to young visually impaired children is that pictures form the base for most preschool stories. Pictures help the story move along in a logical sequence. They serve as guideposts for the story-teller. Pictures also attract the child's attention and help keep his interest. When the child cannot easily see the pictures the story-teller may feel inhibited.

Stories are a form of communication and here lies another problem! Communication is based on a give-and-receive system. We all know how hard it is to talk to a person buried behind a newspaper. There is no eye contact and no response or perhaps just a mumble. There can also be the added frustration when, after a few seconds of silence, the person behind the paper says, 'What is that you said?'

Similar problems, although not for the same reason, can arise when telling a story to a visually impaired child. There may be no eye contact and the child may appear uninterested. In group situations he may even have his back to the speaker. This is confusing for the person looking for a response, and the confusion is understandable because much of our communication is through eye contact and gestures. Facial expressions help indicate how the words are being received. When the child is looking away or his face is expressionless, it can be very disconcerting.

Words, our major form of communication, frequently have visual connotations; they form a picture in one's mind. Preschoolers are still learning about words. For the sighted preschooler the process is quicker. Words are visually reinforced on a daily basis. The blind preschooler may need extra time to process words into non-visual terms and therefore may be a little slower in responding to the story-teller. A lack of response or a different response from what is expected is a difficulty that can arise very early, often when the child is still an infant.

Consider a parent with a small child on his or her knee. She points to a picture or an object and makes a simple statement about it: 'Look at the pretty kitty. Meow! Kitty is talking to you. Look how soft she is.' Or 'See the picture of the pretty flower. It's a big, yellow flower.' The child may be too young to verbally communicate, but the mother is usually rewarded by a smile, gurgle, or a small hand reaching out.

The parent of a visually impaired or multihandicapped child does not get this response. Spontaneously he or she may point to a kitten and say, 'Look! Nice kitty.' There may be no obvious reaction from the small child, so the parent picks up the kitten and takes the child's hand to feel it. There still may be no reaction, or the child may show interest, surprise, or perhaps fear. Whatever the response, it will be different from that of a fully sighted child and is seldom as rewarding to the parent. It is not surprising if, after a while, the parent's spontaneous chatter to the child decreases or completely stops. With the parent's natural spontaneity stifled, communication can become stilted or forced and story-telling seems difficult, if thought of at all.

Another barrier is the knowledge that the child should have words accompanied by concrete experiences. Professionals in the field frequently remind parents not to confuse the child with unnecessary details or meaningless jingles, and to keep their statements factual so that the child can relate to what is said and have a correct understanding of the words. Parents understand the reason for these instructions. As stories are frequently fantasy, it seems difficult to equate them with concrete experiences. Consequently, story-telling may not be thought of as an appropriate activity for a visually impaired child.

It is often difficult to find a book that matches the child's non-visual understanding of his world and is in keeping with his limited experience. Certainly some stories can be adapted, but that is not always easy to do. No great harm and indeed some good can be derived from listening to stories that are not totally meaningful. However, such stories can cause confusion and may stop the child from trying to makes sense of the words he hears. In spite of the barriers, story-telling can be fun and is appropriate for the visually impaired, non-verbal, or multihandicapped child.

Benefits of Story-telling

Hearing stories can foster a feeling of togetherness. There is the pleasure of being in another's company, and the sound of a voice can be soothing. If started early, story-telling can help even the most restless child to relax, be still, and listen. For visually impaired children, these three skills are very difficult but necessary, especially for the child soon to be attending nursery school or kindergarten.

Stories help to exercise memory. This is of particular importance to the visually impaired or multihandicapped child who cannot easily explore his world and does not have the constant visual reinforcement to jog his memory. Stories help the child organize his thoughts regarding daily events and casual experiences. Within the framework of the story, information that may have been missed can be added. Through story-telling new experiences can be introduced, such as a birthday party or a visit to the dentist.

Words do become meaningful for the blind child, but some words will take much longer to be fully understood. This is especially true for the multihandicapped child, whose opportunities for experiential learning may be limited. As the words are repeated many times through the story, the child becomes familiar with them. Stories can overcome disturbing experiences.

A totally blind child, who had been adopted, was very frightened by the sound of a baby crying. Her parents had no idea what their new daughter associated with the sound. Taking Stella into any public place became a traumatic experience because babies can be heard crying almost everywhere! If they were to lead a normal life, Stella had to overcome her real fear of the sound of an infant crying. Story-telling was the method her parents used to help her. They started by imitating noises, including the noise of a baby crying, and in a short while they had made the imitation of the noise into a fun experience. In fact, they used the crying noise in much the same way as a hug or a tickle. The family adapted and made up stories about babies. They then introduced Stella to a tiny, happy baby. A real baby not a doll, although they used dolls to illustrate rocking and cuddling while the story unfolded. In a few months through stories and a planned progression of events, Stella understood babies and learned not to fear a baby's cry. Weaning Stella from the fun of the loud, pretend crying noise took much longer!

A story can be fanciful yet express concrete ideas. If the fantasy is built on objects and experiences that are familiar, it can develop imagination and give new understanding. We don't always have objects to touch or pictures to point to when we talk. For the visually impaired child we can build a word picture that matches his non-visual understanding of the world. For example, 'The cookie was round and rough. Ian could feel the bumps of the chocolate chips. He liked the smell of the cookie and the sound of the crunch when he bit into it with his teeth. The chocolate chips tasted sweet on his tongue.'

Most communication is based on day-to-day events. For small children, stories built on daily experiences are most effective. There is always a base to build on, regardless of how disabled the child may be. Sleeping, eating, dressing, or any number of normal events in the child's day can become topics in a fun story.

If you watch people when they are relaxed and enjoying conversation, you will see that their faces, body gestures, and voice inflections are an integral part of their conversation, and so it should be when story-telling. Voice inflection is a key to success. A simple statement can have a variety of meanings, depending on how it is said. 'I love you' can be passionate, romantic, or affectionate. It can express light-hearted teasing, frustration, or sarcasm. Remembering this is important as visually impaired children miss most facial expressions and body gestures that highlight and enhance the meaning of the words they hear. Conscious attention to voice inflection can help replace what has been missed. For the child with very limited vision, exaggerate facial expression and gestures and encourage the child to imitate you.

Our voices can add interest and can be likened in many ways to a whole orchestra. A voice can be melodious or lilting, go fast or slow, hum, chant, whistle or sing, be deep or high-pitched, and produce any number of interesting sounds. Preschoolers and young children love different sounds!

Be creative with your voice and whenever possible encourage the child to participate. Listen to the sounds your children make when they are drinking their milk, splashing in the bath, whimpering or whining, roaring in anger, giggling or laughing. Imitate these sounds. These can be the equivalent of pictures and just as much fun for the visually impaired child. Also include environmental sounds, such as the lapping sound the dog makes when drinking his water, the baby's rattle, dad shaving, scissors cutting, coats being zipped, wind and rain, car on the gravel. Your voice may not duplicate the sounds, but there can be a similarity. When the child hears the real sound, you can remind him of his story or vice versa.

Although stories can increase vocabulary and refine and develop language into something beautiful and a joy to listen to, early stories for the visually impaired child must be in a language the child is familiar with and hears on a daily basis. Only after the basic meaning of the story is fully understood should new and unfamiliar words be introduced. It is important to remember that your initial goal should be to enjoy communicating with your child. All other learning is a natural progression from this.

Finally, repetition is what will make your story a winner! Little children love to hear the same stories retold, as well as repetition within a story.

> Three preschoolers were staying with their aunt. On the first night she put on a tape with a short story. The children enjoyed it. On the next night she was looking for something different, but the children's voices stopped her. 'Can't we hear what we had last night?' they asked. Each night for a full week the children insisted on the same story. What amazed their aunt most was that their enthusiasm grew with each successive hearing. They began to giggle, then laugh outright before the story-teller had even finished the point. To her surprise the youngest, who was just beginning to speak, began repeating some of the words along with the story-teller.

Repetition within the story is also important because it allows the child to anticipate and, when ready, participate. This is especially important for the young visually impaired or multihandicapped child, who may have more difficulty integrating and understanding information than the sighted child. As a potential story-teller you may think repetition sounds very boring. Looking at it from a more positive point of view, repetition means you don't need a whole repertoire of stories. You need only one or two, then build on a few familiar experiences, and these will become the favourites. Small children are easy to please!

Use objects and actions to enhance your story. Some story-tellers like to have something to show the child as they proceed through the story. If you want to do this, we suggest you collect items and keep them handy. A shoe box or cookie tin works well. You never know when your preschoolers are going to say, 'Tell me the story about ...' Once an object has been introduced, not having it available would be like having a story with the 'good' part missing! The most effective items are those that are small enough for the child's hands to explore quickly. Avoid items that have a great deal of detail, as the child may be trying to decide what it is he is feeling and miss some of the story. If you stop to discuss what he has in his hands, you may lose the continuity. Small items that have a familiar fragrance or sound can also be effective. You can even have something to taste or smell if it fits your story. As you tell the story, briefly place the items in the child's hands, or pass the fragrance close to his nose. Do not force the child to touch, smell, or taste if he is unwilling to do so.

The actions within your story are as important as repetition. Keep the actions simple, and be sure they follow your story-line. We want you to have a wonderful time with your child. Start by telling very short stories until you feel confident. The following are simple stories that you might like to adapt to suit your child and family. As previously suggested, you could use a box or cookie tin to store the items you choose to use. Like sighted children, visually impaired children like to have books of their own. You can make the following story into a book. (See Chapter 5.)

A Morning-Time Story

This story is based on a short time period in the child's day. It has a simple song that can be sung to a child or later by the child to his parent or friend.

Cover: Insert the words and music for the 'Good Morning' song.

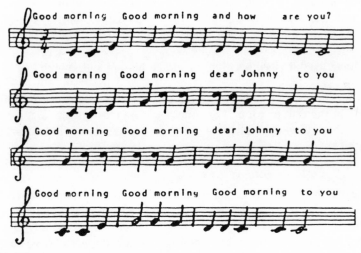

First page
    I am sitting on Mummy's knee
    I feel her arm close 'round me
    This is where I like to be

Sitting on my Mummy's knee.
Very soon we will look
At my special story-book.
Here are my fingers
And this is my thumb.
With these, I'll turn the pages
One by one.
Mummy and I will have such fun.

(If not mother, change 'Mummy' to the name of the reader. A gentle squeeze, a touch of the child's hand on the story-teller's knee, a raised knee to indicate lap. Briefly put the book to the child's hands, touching fingers and thumb. The older child can turn a page.)

Second page

I knew a little boy and his name was Johnny, just like you. One day Johnny woke up, put out his hand and found his rattle. He knew he was in his own crib. Johnny wanted his Mummy, so he made a little noise to let her know he was awake. He listened and heard her footsteps coming. As she bent down to pick him up, he smelled her nice perfume.

Mummy gave him a big hug, and a kiss right on the end of his nose. She said, 'Good morning, Johnny. How are you today?' 'Shall we sing our "Good Morning" song like Mummy sings it?' (*Sing 'Good Morning' song.*)

Johnny liked it when his Mummy picked him up and sang to him.

(Use the child's own name. Rattle can be replaced by anything familiar in the crib or room. Perfume could be face-cream, talc, face-powder, etc. Use unwashed jars for fragrance. Hug and kiss as indicated.)

Third page

Johnny heard somebody coming and knew it was his Daddy. Daddy took Johnny in his strong arms and gave him a big hug and two little kisses on his left cheek and one on his right cheek. Johnny could smell Daddy's shaving-cream. Daddy had just shaved his face, and it was a nice smell.

Daddy said, 'Good morning, Johnny. How are you today? Shall we sing our "Good Morning" song like Daddy sings it?' (*Sing 'Good Morning' song.*)

Johnny liked it when his Daddy sang to him and swung him high in the air, like this. 'I have to go to work,' said Daddy. 'Bye, Johnny. Can you wave your hand goodbye to me?'

(Shaving-cream can be hair tonic, soap, etc. Do actions as indicated.)

Fourth page

Johnny heard another person coming to his room, and he knew it was Susie. Susie was small and she gave him a little hug and a big kiss on his forehead. Johnny could smell toothpaste. Susie had just cleaned her teeth and it was a nice smell.

Susie said, 'Good morning, Johnny. How are you today? Shall we sing our "Good Morning" song like Susie sings it?' (*Sing 'Good Morning' song.*)

Mummy told Susie to hurry or she would be late for school. 'Bye, Johnny,' said Susie, waving her hand. 'Can you wave your hand good-bye to me?'

(Use an empty toothpaste tube for fragrance. Touch the child's teeth. Do other actions as indicated.)

Fifth page

Mummy told Johnny it was time to get him bathed and dressed. She took Johnny to the bathroom and he could smell the soap. She put him in the tub and washed him all over. She washed his eyes, she washed his nose, she washed his mouth, and behind his ears.

Then she washed all over his face. Next, she did his neck and his tummy and all the way down to his knees, and then right on down to the tips of his toes. When she washed his toes, it tickled and made Johnny laugh.

Then his Mummy turned him over and washed his back. After this, she took him out of the tub and rubbed him dry with his soft towel.

Johnny didn't want to come out of the tub, so he cried (*imitate crying*), but when his Mummy rubbed his tummy and jiggled him on her knees, he laughed (*imitate laughter*). Then his Mummy dressed him and he was ready for breakfast. Downstairs they went. Johnny was now ready for a new day!

(Touch all body parts as mentioned. Soap could be talc, oil, etc. Use a large towel and wrap around him briefly as the story unfolds. The older child can touch a piece of towel attached by one edge to the page. Tickle the child's toes (if he enjoys it), jiggle him, and encourage laughter. You could also enlarge on the idea of dressing, listing clothes and touching body parts in the order the clothes would be put on.)

Last page
  Now the story is all done.
  Thank you, Mummy, that was fun.
  Here is a kiss, and a hug too,
  Because dear Mummy, I love you.

(An older child can say the rhyme with the reader. Each says the other's name, e.g., Mummy says 'Johnny' and Johnny says 'Mummy,' and they exchange hugs and kisses.)

A Lunch-Time Story

Here is an outline for a simple story about a familiar activity. In this situation it reinforces self-feeding with appropriate language. Although it is short and simple, it provides an opportunity for using all your story-telling techniques. Use it as a guide for making up your own story or adapt this one to your situation.

It was lunch-time. Katie could smell the food and hear Mummy getting the dishes out of the cupboard. Katie was feeling very hungry. When Mummy put the dish on her tray, Katie held the dish with her left hand and took the spoon with her right hand. Katie curled her *thumb* and her *fingers* around the *handle* of the spoon. She put the spoon in the dish and said, 'Dip, slide, and into my mouth.' Katie opened her mouth very wide and in went the spoon with some _____ (*name food*). Mmmm, it tasted good. Katie swallowed the _____ (*name food*) and it went *all the way down* to her tummy (*do actions*). It was so good. Yum! Yum!
  (*Repeat with two different foods.*)
  Soon Katie wasn't hungry anymore. Mummy said, 'You have finished. Your food has all gone.' Katie put her fingers in the dish and said, 'It's all gone.' Mummy wiped Katie's hands and lifted her down. Katie ran off to play.

Judy Loses Her Ice-cream

Every week Judy and her mother went grocery shopping. This week they bought bread in the bakery section of the supermarket. Next they came to the fruit and vegetables. Judy helped her mother put apples and oranges in a bag. Mother said, 'Shall we buy a cantaloupe to eat with our ice-cream?' Judy said, 'No. I just like ice-cream.' Next they picked out some vegetables, then on to the canned foods, meat, and dairy sections of the store.

Judy helped her mother push the cart to the check-out counter. As they got close to the counter Judy could hear the noise of the cash register and her mother said, 'There are three people ahead of us; we will have to wait.' As they waited, Judy asked, 'Mummy, are we going to the ice-cream shop next?' 'Yes, we always do that. What flavour would you like today?' 'I like vanilla best' said Judy. 'I hoped you would surprise me and choose something different today,' laughed her mother.

After the groceries were paid for and put into bags, Judy helped her mother carry them out to the car and off they went to the ice-cream shop.

Mrs. Graydon was behind the counter and said, 'Good morning, Judy.' 'Hi, Mrs Graydon,' Judy said. 'How nice, you remembered my name,' said Mrs Graydon. 'What flavour would you like today?' 'Vanilla,' Judy said quickly. Mrs Graydon said, 'I have some different flavours you could try: strawberry, orange-licorice, and chocolate chip.' She handed Judy a small plastic spoon with a little strawberry ice-cream on it. Judy tasted it and said, 'Mmmmm. But I like vanilla best.' Next Mrs Graydon handed her a small plastic spoon with a little orange-licorice ice-cream on it. Judy tasted it and said 'Mmmmm. That tastes different, but I like vanilla best.' Then Mrs Graydon handed her a small plastic spoon with a little chocolate chip ice-cream on it. Judy tasted it, licked her lips and said, 'Mmmmm, that's good.' 'So what flavour will you choose today?' Judy's mother asked. Judy thought for a moment and then said, 'I'll surprise you. I would like chocolate chip today.' Her mother said, 'Well, well. Hip hip hooray! We'll have chocolate chip today!'

When they got home Judy said, 'May I have some ice-cream right now?' Her mother said, 'I'll put some in a dish for you before I put the groceries away.'

Judy hurried to the washroom. When she had finished, she flushed the toilet and washed and dried her hands. When she got to the door, she felt she would like to flush the toilet just once more. Judy liked the sound of the toilet flushing. Then she remembered her ice-cream and hurried to the kitchen. 'Mummy, where's my ice-cream?' 'I put it on the table for you. It's in the glass dish with the bumpy pattern that you like so much.' Judy went to the table and found the glass dish and the spoon Mummy had put beside it. Judy put her spoon into the dish, but she didn't find any ice-cream. She put her spoon in again and still she didn't find any ice-cream. So she put her fingers in the dish. She didn't find any ice-cream and her fingers were all wet. Judy said, 'This is not like the ice-cream Mrs Graydon gave me.' Judy was very disappointed.

Judy's mother came to the table and began to laugh. Why was her mother laughing? Judy didn't think it was funny. She had been looking forward to this new taste. Judy sounded cross. She said, 'I wish I had asked for vanilla.'

Judy's mother stopped laughing and said, 'This is like the ice-cream that Mrs Graydon let you taste, but this ice-cream has melted. You asked for your ice-cream right now but you took a long time in the washroom and it is warm in the kitchen. Never mind, I'll give you another dish of ice-cream.'

Judy's mother went to the freezer and scooped more ice-cream out of the container and put it in a clean dish for Judy. She said, 'See if it tastes like the ice-cream Mrs Graydon let you taste.' Judy put in her spoon and felt the firm ice-cream and put some in her mouth. She said, 'This is like the ice-cream Mrs Graydon let me taste. Mmmmmmm, it's good.' Judy's mother said, 'You'd better eat it quickly if you don't want it to melt again.'

Judy enjoyed her ice-cream. She didn't know that ice-cream melted so quickly. Judy's mother said, 'Ice-cream is a bit like cold snow. It melts when it is warm. Remember when you and Daddy made snow-balls and Daddy's melted in his hands?' Judy remembered, then said, 'I don't like melted ice-cream.'

(Point out other things that melt: chocolate in warm pockets, butter left out of the fridge on a hot day, ice in a drink. Also things that can be frozen: juice into popsicles, water into ice-cubes, sandwiches for tomorrow's picnic.)

NINE

Nursery School and Kindergarten

In Canada in the 1950s, a few nursery schools became receptive to experimentally enrolling visually impaired children in their schools, mainly through the efforts of people working with young blind and partially sighted children. The idea spread and now visually impaired children can be found in various programs with their sighted peers. In today's society with many parents working, enrolling a visually impaired child in a community program is the norm rather than the exception. However, enrolment does need careful consideration.

Parents and educators still have questions and concerns about whether it is appropriate to have a visually impaired child in nursery school with fully sighted children. Their apprehension and confusion are natural, for while enrolment in community programs is normal, visual impairment in children is not. In this section we offer a few suggestions to make a smooth transition from home to nursery school.

Special Assistance

The nursery school or junior kindergarten experience is extremely important for a young visually impaired child. If he enters the program when he is ready, he should not need someone working solely with him. As a shy, sighted child may need additional time before he is ready to participate fully in the program, so will the visually impaired child who is learning to depend on himself.

When there are large groups of children in nursery school and kindergarten, it will be helpful to have an extra adult. All the children should understand that this person is the teacher's assistant, not the visually impaired child's special helper. The assistant can be helpful, especially in kindergarten, adapting material to meet the visually impaired child's needs, giving the teacher time to work with all the individual children in the group who have special needs.

This nursery school period provides opportunities for the visually impaired child to develop his skills of dependence on self. Following nursery school, the visually impaired child will be receiving formal education that will require increased individual help if his educational needs are to be fully met. Extra help may be essential, but unless the child has developed confidence, understands how to be on his own, and operates independently as one of the group, he may transfer his dependence on his family to his special teacher.

Segregated Settings

Few visually impaired children are fortunate enough to live close to a preschool program designed especially for them. Such a setting offers support for parents and gives a child the opportunity to become comfortable in a new setting and familiar with nursery school routines. It will also provide opportunities for the child to learn in his own way, and at his own pace, the basic concepts, as well as language, listening, socialization, and daily living skills that will prepare him as early and as fully as possible for integration into the sighted world. This is an excellent beginning, but you should make sure your child also has a regular opportunity to meet and interact confidently with sighted preschoolers (e.g., Sunday School, swim group). Why send a visually impaired child to nursery school?

- to prepare for formal education
- to provide an opportunity for parent and child to become comfortable with separation and to give the child a feeling of independence
- to enable the mother to have a break from the demands of meeting the needs of her visually impaired child
- to allow for greater conceptual development through peer interaction in new and challenging experiences
- to learn through free exploration and directed activities how to operate in a peer group situation
- to learn acceptable and effective ways of interacting with peers
- to improve listening skills and the ability to follow directions

- to promote continued development of receptive and expressive language
- to increase attention span
- to improve visual efficiency through the need to use vision in a stimulating and changing environment
- to further develop skills of orientation, exploration, and mobility
- to increase tactual awareness through effective use of the hands
- to develop greater independence in all areas
- to increase opportunities for gross- and fine-motor development
- to help the child become an accepted member of his community
- to provide a positive setting in which the child has an early opportunity to become aware of his similarities to and differences from others, and with this new awareness maintain and continue to develop the foundations of a positive self-image
- to promote continued development of the concept of male and female to further the child's understanding of the words 'boy' and 'girl,' thus enabling the child to identify with his or her own gender

When Is the Child Ready?

Visually impaired children vary considerably in their eye conditions, visual efficiency, personality, intelligence, and the opportunities and experiences they have had. The following are only guidelines to give the reader some indication of what to look for in determining whether a visually impaired child will benefit from an integrated nursery school experience. The first six points are certainly necessary if the child is blind and not multihandicapped.

- understands and responds to own name
- has an awareness of body parts and, on request, can identify or indicate some
- is able to follow simple directions and communicate basic needs
- knows the home routine
- is ambulatory and has some basic living skills
- if not completely toilet-trained, has some understanding of the process
- has a fair knowledge of his home environment and, on request, can locate furniture and rooms
- anticipates events by associating some sounds, smells, and actions
- preferably has had some contact with other children, such as a brother or sister, a Sunday School class, or a local play group

- has heard the term 'blind' or 'visually impaired' in relation to himself

Ideally, the blind child should be considerably further advanced than suggested by the above points. If the child is not ready, consider keeping him at home for a longer period or, if this is not possible, look for an 'in-home' special program.

What to Look For in a Nursery School

- A happy, relaxed atmosphere.
- Teachers who see parents as part of the team.
- Friendly, interested, and experienced teachers.
- School personnel who make cooperation and courtesy a habit.
- Teachers who give children firm and sensitive guide-lines and have realistic behavioural expectations for them.
- Creativity and flexibility in programming.
- Equipment and space both indoors and outdoors that allow for freedom of movement and for the development of fine- and gross-motor skills.
- Sensible arrangement and organization of equipment to ensure maximum safety.
- General cleanliness and a cheerful appearance.
- Well-cared-for equipment and toys.
- Noise level that does not overwhelm the child, and the availability of quiet areas when needed.
- The availability of correct lighting to meet the specific needs of the child as determined by his eye condition. Certain eye conditions necessitate bright, direct lighting, while others require more subdued light. Glare should always be eliminated.

There is not always a choice of nursery schools. If the nursery school in your area does not meet your criteria, it would be wise to consider other alternatives, such as joining with other parents and taking turns in running small neighbourhood play groups. With a little thought and good planning, these can be very successful.

How Can a Blind Child Be Prepared for Nursery School?

Once parents have decided that their child will benefit from nursery school, they can prepare the child by:

- Talking positively to the child about nursery school.
- Reading, making up, or play-acting simple stories about nursery school, stressing various aspects of school activities and comparing them with experiences that the child is already familiar with and understands.
- Exploring playground equipment and comparing it with equipment found in the nursery school.
- Being sure the child has been introduced to neighbourhood children.
- Walking with siblings to and from their school.
- Attending Sunday School, library, 'Mums and Tots' programs, or other activity groups for young children.
- Contacting and arranging a visit to the nursery school when school is not in session so that the child can meet the teacher and explore the facility at his own pace. Some visually impaired children may need several visits, while others may need only one.
- Taking the child to visit the school when in session, but making no demands on the child to be actively involved.
- Taking the child to nursery school and leaving for short periods, gradually lengthening these periods until the child is confident and anticipates the next visit with pleasure. For a blind child, consecutive days are preferable to alternate days. Blocks of time are less confusing and offer greater continuity.

How Can the Nursery School Prepare for a Blind Child?

- By contacting a local agency for the blind to obtain literature and information. By reading literature pertaining to blind children in general.
- By arranging a visit, preferably with both parents present, in order to share information. The teacher will need to know the child's eye condition, what residual vision he has and how this affects his general functioning; any other medical problems the child has, such as food allergies; the child's present level of functioning; activities that give the child the most pleasure; particular dislikes or fears that the child may have; the level of the child's awareness regarding his handicap; familiar vocabulary the child uses for common objects and daily activities; names the child uses for immediate family, relatives, friends, and family pets; who lives in the family home, daily routine, special interest, etc.; any previous group experiences the child has had. Agencies for the blind

usually have trained staff capable of assessing functional vision and advising on ways to help the child increase his visual efficiency.

- By arranging a school visit for the parents and the child when the school is not in session to meet the child and observe his interaction with parents and note their effective ways of helping him; show the child the nursery school and note any special interests he may have that will help in planning for him; observe how comfortable the child is with the equipment and note any difficulties that he encounters; observe how well the child uses his hands for exploring the environment.

- By choosing the permanent reference points to be used in orientating the child to the classroom. Repeated planned exploration of the area will be necessary before the child will be familiar with the layout.

- By deciding if classmates need information to understand the child's visual impairment; for example, the child may have noticeable physical differences, as in some glaucoma cases.

- By ensuring that the classroom teacher feels comfortable about having the child in her room. This is important as her feelings can significantly influence the attitudes of all the children. Initial apprehension is to be expected.

- By informing all members of the staff of any special needs the visually impaired child may have.

- By inviting the parents and the child for a visit when the school is in session. Aim to make this a comfortable experience for all concerned by welcoming the child and the parents and exchanging names; not pressing the child to be involved, but offering him the opportunity; encouraging the other children to talk to him and invite him to play; arranging with the parents times for gradual integration into the program.

Orientating the Child to the Program

Before a blind child can be expected to participate in group activities, he must have several days of individual orientation to the physical layout and routines. Some children will feel more secure if given the opportunity to spend time in one area, for example, the playhouse centre, before gradually being introduced to the total program. For less confident children, several weeks in one area may be necessary. Just as a shy or immature child may prefer the security of one spot until, through observation, he is comfortable with the program, so too the visually impaired child may need time to assess the program through auditory means.

One way to introduce the child to the school layout is to note a few major reference points. These could be the cloakroom, the washroom, and perhaps one or two areas in the classroom in which the child showed particular interest on his initial visit to the school.

Show the child the simplest route from the cloakroom to the favourite area. Do this slowly. Name what he is passing. Do not insist, but give him the opportunity to examine the objects he passes. Remember to use the same route and name the same objects each time. As soon as possible allow the child to find his way independently along the route you have shown him. You may be surprised to find how quickly he will do this if you resist the temptation to help or correct him each time. Be patient. He needs time to practise, and this includes the opportunity to make and correct mistakes. The following are additional points specific to nursery school or kindergarten:

- Choose a coat peg at the beginning or end of a row. Use a tactual or auditory marker for easy identification. If children have individual chairs or equipment, use a similar marker for these. If the child is blind, you may want to consider putting his name in braille. Do not try to teach him the letters, just let him experience the feel. The sighted children will be interested too.
- It is important for the parent and the teacher to share information on a regular basis. A daily logbook passed between the parent and the teacher is helpful in recording the child's special interests and activities of the day. Remember to add some little details. Language development is increased through conversation that is meaningful to the visually impaired child. If the parent and the teacher discuss daily events with the child, continuity is built and accurate concepts are developed.
- It will be helpful to advise the visually impaired child when furniture or activity centres are changed.
- Sighted children observe events, imitate and compare, and use unrelated objects to act out their ideas. Visually impaired children have limited visual experiences from which to draw and may need help in developing imaginative play.
- Visual impairment should not be an excuse for inappropriate behaviour. However, for a visually impaired child to understand

behaviourial expectations, behaviour must be clearly identified. To do this, it may be necessary to request the child to repeat the unacceptable behaviour and label it. A demonstration of what is acceptable behaviour should follow immediately.

- When a visual clue indicates a change of activity, the visually impaired child will need an auditory clue.
- In periods such as story, circle, or snack time, encourage the children sitting beside a visually impaired child to identify themselves.
- Include the visually impaired child's name in the instructions. This helps the child to learn that he is part of the group and expected to participate.
- The visually impaired child will need some explanation of what the group is doing, especially when it is necessary for him to wait for a slower child, an unexpected event, or a snack to arrive. When a waiting period proves to be lengthy, giving the child a small item to manipulate (e.g., an elastic band or a paper-clip) will help him to compensate for the lack of visual interest.
- The visually impaired child needs to be told when he is keeping the group waiting.

Giving Directions to a Child Individually

Remember to preface directions with the child's name and use simple, explicit language. If the child does not follow the verbal directions, guide him physically through it, then say, 'Let's try again.' Return to the beginning of the situation and repeat the verbal directions. Wait long enough to allow the child time to think over what you have said. If the child still appears not to understand, then give him a physical prompt and again wait for him to try. Be patient. It may take longer for him to respond. If you still do not get results, move on to the next activity and repeat the whole process at a later time. If after several repetitions the child is still not following directions independently, look for hidden stumbling-blocks. It could be due to a number of reasons.

- The child may be conditioned to act only after physical prompts or repeated verbal directions.
- The child is having a problem understanding the words being used.
- The child's level of concept development makes the instructions confusing.

- The child may lack confidence or be afraid.
- The child may be distracted by the sounds and activities around him and therefore not able to concentrate on the instructions.
- The child may be using manipulative behaviour (this is the least likely possibility).

Circle Time

- To help the visually impaired child understand the meaning of sitting in a 'circle,' it is useful initially to walk him around the circle before he is shown his own place. This gives him the idea that all the children are together.
- Seating the visually impaired child close to the teacher or the source of music will assist him to concentrate on the presentation by making other sounds less distracting. However, in determining the most beneficial place for the child to sit, his visual abilities should be considered. Observe the child's choice of seating. His choice may be the most beneficial place for him.
- Give individual instructions for new song actions. This can be done before or during the circle time. The visually impaired child can be involved in demonstrating to the other children. This can be helpful in three ways: while the child is demonstrating, he is also learning the activity; it may give the other children a greater awareness of the visually impaired child's special needs; it can serve to foster a positive self-image in the visually impaired child. Many parents would enjoy teaching the visually impaired child the actions to songs. If teachers write the words out ahead of time and give them to the parents, the child will benefit from the extra practice and enjoy this time with his parent.

Story Time

- Sit the child close to the teacher so her occasional touch can compensate for the eye contact available to the sighted children. Remember that even the active visually impaired child may not be able to make eye contact.
- It is sometimes helpful to allow the visually impaired child to hold the book and turn pages on request as the teacher reads. Providing the child with an active role gives him a feeling of usefulness and increases his level of awareness of the group activity.

- While the story may not be totally relevant to the child's experiences, story time is important for the development of social and listening skills. However, care should be taken to ensure that the child is not too confused. Whenever possible a prior individual introduction to the story with a special explanation from the teacher or the parent will be helpful.

Snack Time

- Expect age-appropriate table manners.
- Encourage all children to identify food and drink by taste and smell.
- Tell the visually impaired child when his snack is in front of him. Allow him to locate it briefly, then expect him to wait with hands in lap if that is the expectation for the group.
- When it is the visually impaired child's turn to pass the cookies, it is a good idea to encourage the sighted children to assist verbally, e.g., 'I'm Peter. I've taken two cookies. John is next.' This not only helps the visually impaired child, but gives the sighted children a better understanding of the visually impaired child's needs and enhances the language development of all the children.

Outdoor Play

Just as orientation to the classroom is necessary before a visually impaired child can be expected to function independently, orientation to the outdoor area is also necessary. Give special attention to reference points that indicate locations for fun, as well as potential danger areas such as swings. Indicators to guide the child can be *auditory* (a windchime on the toy-shed, a bell on the swing), *tactual* (a marker tied on the fence, a piece of garden hose across an open area), different ground *textures* (gravel, grass, pavement), *contours* (a small hill, a pothole).

- Many visually impaired children need peaked caps or sunglasses on sunny days, especially if there is glare from snow or water on the ground.
- Show the blind child how to participate in all activities. This includes taking his turn at pushing or pulling peers in or on mobile toys.
- Give practical demonstrations with verbal explanations of a line-up and of waiting in turn for the slide or the swing.

- Draw the child's attention to outdoor sounds, smells, and textures. Remember, these can also be considered as clues to location.

Free Activity Period

Before a visually impaired child can use the free activity period as constructively as his sighted peers, he needs to be shown what is available and how to use it. He may often need to be reminded of the choices he has. The visually impaired child should make his own choices. If he always chooses the same activity, determine whether this is his preference or whether he has forgotten the options.

A blind child will sometimes ask to paint. This is not as strange as it may seem. Most activities require great concentration for the blind child and may prevent him from interacting with his peers. Painting is relaxing, repetitious, and may be a meaningless movement for the blind child requiring little concentration. It may provide an opportunity for him to direct his energies into conversing with his peers.

If in fact it is a free play period (in some schools this period has some structure), wandering around the room and exploring is an appropriate activity for the visually impaired child. Guard against redirecting him too quickly. His wanderings may not be as aimless as they appear. He may be gaining information through his non-visual senses.

On occasion, the free activity period could be used to explain parts of the story he will hear later that may be unfamiliar to him. It could also be used to teach him the actions of a new song. He could help the teacher prepare for a new activity, thus increasing the general knowledge that he cannot obtain by observation.

Braille or Print?

Whether your child is to be a braille or print user, many of the activities in nursery school and kindergarten are preparation for reading. This includes sorting, stringing beads randomly or following a pattern, cutting, pasting, puzzles, and all fine-motor activities. Concept development is also part of reading readiness. Story-telling and role-playing in the activity centres help develop concepts.

Unless the child is blind, it will sometimes be difficult to determine whether braille or print will be the medium he uses to read. Many factors influence visual functioning, including personality and motivation. A professional who is skilled in functional vision testing will be able to help you decide which medium is best for your child.

TEN

Preventive and Remedial Measures

When problems arise, having a knowledgeable professional to advise you is always helpful, but sometimes they are just not available when you need them most! Remedial approaches can be found for almost any problem if you have enough basic knowledge, keep an open mind, and are willing to patiently think it through. In this section, we will try to give you further insight and practical guides to help you prevent or solve some of the simple or complex problems you may encounter. The section also addresses issues relating to confused and emotionally fragile children. If you use it in conjunction with the rest of the book, you may discover that your most valuable professional is you; the others are your helpmates along the road.

The Learning Process

The way a visually impaired child learns and builds information is often likened to the solving of a jigsaw puzzle, which must be fitted together before the whole is understood. This is a good analogy, but does not emphasize the crumbling effect when several pieces of information are missing from a child's basic knowledge. This crumbling effect can be seen in very confused children who function below their potential and who may even exhibit deviant behaviour. Frequently it is due to large gaps in a child's basic information, making his world confusing and meaningless.

Instead of a flat puzzle, we will use the analogy of a transparent puzzle ball. This transparent ball, like a rolling snowball, can grow increasingly larger. It can become firm in the centre, or it can have lumps and be misshapen; it may even crumble. At the centre of this puzzle ball is a solid coloured piece representing the child. The ball is made up of transparent, slightly flexible layers, each layer overlapping another and representing a total concept. If a child is sighted, each layer consists of information gathered by touch, sound, smell, and taste, and then put together through vision into one transparent whole representing an understood concept or idea.

For the visually impaired child, the puzzle ball is formed in the same way, layer upon layer; however, there is a major difference – *the layers are in pieces.* Without the sighted child's ability to visually – and often at a glance – integrate information, the visually impaired child's information is fragmented, and every separate piece must be carefully fitted together before each layer can be formed.

Unlike that of the sighted infant, the visually impaired infant's world is as far as his body reaches, which includes what he hears, as well as what he feels, tastes, or smells, and, if he has any vision, what little he is able to see. These sensory contacts make up pieces of a layer.

The large pieces of the first layer represent information relating to the child, his mother, and other primary caregivers, usually his family. The smaller pieces in between represent information about all inanimate things – clothing, toys, furniture, activities, etc. These small pieces must be connected to the larger pieces to fill in the spaces between the visually impaired child and the key people in his world. When the first layer – self, family, and home – is fitted firmly together, it forms the first basic concepts on which each additional layer will be built. With correctly completed layers, the centre becomes firmly packed and gradually solidified. It is on this solid base, formed primarily during the preschool years, that all other information and formal education must be built. For the visually impaired child, this process is long. It is this solidifying or crumbling action that is so important and perhaps overlooked in the flat jigsaw analogy.

Information is gathered and then processed into an idea or thought. If it stays at this stage, it is tentative and fragile. If a child is exposed to new information or experiences, the idea or thought may become solidified as a proved or disproved fact. Left in the tentative stage, it can remain a mystery to the child and cause confusion. For example, Mr Barber, hurrying down the hall, glances casually into the living-room and sees a woman's back that he doesn't immediately recognize. He thinks a friend of his wife must be visiting, but hurries on. The idea or thought is formed but tentative. A few minutes later, he hears a woman's voice from the living-room. It sounds like his sister-in-law whom he hasn't seen for a while. The idea or thought is taking shape, but it is not yet confirmed. Mr Barber goes back to the living-room and finds his wife and a neighbour, not his sister-in-law, but notes the similarity in their voices. Now the idea is confirmed. There are no questions; it is solid information. His wife and the neighbour are visiting. For the visually impaired child, experiences with people and objects may have to be repeated many times for them to become confirmed facts.

Now, imagine being able to look through to the very centre of the transparent puzzle ball. If you see many pieces missing, you will know that unless those pieces are inserted, the ball will crumble when new layers are added. Look again and you may notice the solid area is not as it should be – a fully rounded, solidified centre – but rather isolated lumps with missing pieces all around, perhaps attached to incomplete layers above or below. These solid lumps represent skills or understood information that has not been accurately connected and therefore cannot be utilized in a meaningful way by the child. In some cases, the total ball will appear to be crumbling. In others, it is wavy and out of shape, and unless the pieces are put in place and are all connected, new information only adds to the crumbling effect.

When the visually impaired child has difficulty in learning, it is usually due to missing pieces or pieces placed incorrectly. When problems are increasing, then the foundation may be crumbling. When the child seems to be on a plateau, there may be lumps with the connections missing. Whatever the cause, remedial action must be taken and, if necessary, must reach right to the foundation. The non-visual perspective is the tool kit that can locate and cement the missing pieces. Without it, only Band-Aid solutions are possible.

The *non-visual perspective* is looking at the situation from a non-visual point of view, putting yourself in the visually impaired child's place. Throughout the book we have emphasized the non-visual perspective, but more than superficial attention must be paid to it in order to understand the uniqueness of the visually impaired child. Taste, smell, sound, limited vision – each in its own right could be a focus for the non-visual perspective. Because physical contact is so important, we have chosen to focus on touch for this exploration.

Touch is a form of communication and, like words, can sometimes be confusing. Unless the non-visual perspective is used, the root cause of the confusion may not be understood. In this next situation, see if you can recognize the cause of Freddie's problem.

Freddie had no vision. Every week he accompanied his mother when she did the grocery shopping. His mother would bring the bags of groceries from the car and Freddie opened the latch-type door.

When Freddie was eight years old the family moved to a new home. As before, after the shopping expedition Freddie went to open the door, but this time the handle needed to be turned. 'This door opens differently,' his mother said. 'Turn the handle, Freddie.' But Freddie had no success. Putting her parcels down, Freddie's mother showed him how to turn the handle. As she instructed him with her hand over his she said, 'You turn it, not press down as you did on our old door.' With the next bag of groceries, Freddie again went to open the door, but still had no success.

'Turn,' his mother said, 'you know how to turn it, I have just shown you.' But Freddie still was not able to open the door. 'For Pete's sake,' his mother said in frustration, 'turn it the way you wind your old music box.' Immediately Freddie opened the door.

One would suppose that by eight years of age Freddie had come across doors with handles that turned, so why was Freddie not opening the door? Perhaps in other situations the doors had always been open, or someone had opened them for him. Could it be that he didn't understand the word 'turn'? Yet his mother had shown him hand over hand what 'turn' meant, so that wouldn't appear to be the problem. At the word 'wind,' Freddie opened the door immediately, suggesting that 'wind' and not 'turn' was the word he understood. But then why had the hand-over-hand method not helped? Surely that would be the concrete way to *show* him what 'turn' meant? Some people might conclude that Freddie is being stubborn or uncooperative, or that he is intellectually impaired.

Freddie was confused by the word 'turn,' not because he didn't understand the word, but because he was blind. The most frequently used meaning for the word 'turn' was a full body movement – turn to the right or left, turn around, etc. The word 'turn' and his mother's hand over his were not giving the same message. If he had vision, Freddie could have seen what 'turn' meant.

You probably recognized Freddie's problem. His confusion is

common to all of us from time to time. We can easily become confused momentarily or even for long periods by something that is totally uncomplicated and straightforward to another person. The reason is usually quite simple. We have arrived at the experience, situation, or statement from a different reference point and at the moment our reference point and the new information do not have the same meaning. When the confusion clears, we wonder how we could have been so stupid! Playing on people's different reference points or understanding is often a basis for jokes and comedy. However, it is not comical for the visually impaired child when he is confused and when those who interact with him jump to the wrong conclusion and do not use the non-visual perspective to try to determine his reference point.

To appreciate the significance of touch – skin against skin – it is necessary to really think about the role vision plays in what a sighted person understands when he is touched. It is very easy to misinterpret a blind child's actions or reactions when they differ from what might be expected. The message a blind child receives from the touch of skin against skin is frequently the message intended. However, when the response is unusual or unexpected, there is only one thing that is certain: *a message has been received but, without the help of vision, it has been misinterpreted.* Consider the following situations.

Sally was a totally blind six-year-old. She had been delayed in walking. Although she now had caught up, her parents used every method they could use to help her strengthen her muscles and use her legs. In the playroom there was a slide designed for a much younger child. On this occasion Sally was being challenged to pull herself up. She had been instructed to lie on her tummy on the slide, her toes just off the floor. Sally was using her arms and legs reciprocally to move herself up the slide. To encourage her, her father said, 'Good pulling, Sally,' and he touched her arm lightly. Immediately Sally relaxed the arm touched, but continued to use her other limbs. Surprised, her father continued, 'Come on, Sally, you are pulling well,' and touched her leg just to emphasize his words. Again the same thing. She relaxed the leg touched but kept her arms and other leg moving. To continue encouraging her, Sally's father touched only her head and Sally, using arms and legs, pulled with increased vigour the rest of the way. Sally's mother was at the top of the slide, her fingers just over the edge. 'Keep coming, Sally,' she said, 'you've almost reached me.' Sally stretched out both her arms for an extra pull and her fingers came in contact with her mother's fingertips. To her parents' amazement, Sally immediately stopped all pulling, but she did not relax. Her head was up and her body poised ready to go, yet she did not make any attempt to move further. Sally's mother did not reach down to her but instead said, 'Sally, you haven't quite reached the top yet. You are just touching my fingers. If you get hold of my hands I'll help you.' But Sally did not move. Her father said, 'Use your arms, Sally, and pull a little more.' Sally did.

Why did Sally stop moving an individual limb each time she felt her father's touch? Why did she stop altogether when in contact with her mother's fingertips? What was the difference between her mother's words and those of her father? Or was it their combined instructions that made Sally move again? What is the significance of skin against skin?

Philip had only light perception. He was born prematurely. Although alert and bright with good receptive language and some expressive language, his self-help skills were delayed. Philip was three-and-a-half years old, but had not fully mastered using his spoon to feed himself and needed help dressing and undressing. Philip had been receiving help from a special needs worker, a person hired to give Philip individual help to catch up. This person had worked hard to help him. She had used the hand-over-hand method to show Philip how to use the spoon, but he would let go of the spoon as soon as her hand was off his.

With great patience his special worker persevered, showing and encouraging until Philip would use the spoon without her hand on his. However, he would not scoop the food onto the spoon unless he felt her hand. So, she lightly placed her hand on his wrist. In a very short time, Philip was doing the whole process very efficiently. Convinced that Philip was now fully confident and had no need for her hand on his wrist, his special worker removed it. Philip paused for a moment, but was encouraged to keep scooping. He did, but not before placing his own free hand on his wrist; in this awkward position, he continued to feed himself. His worker watched in total disbelief.

What was the significance of his worker's touch? Why did Philip put his own hand on his wrist when this position made feeding himself awkward? Although not common, Philip's is not an isolated case.

Three-year-old Roderick loved nursery school and especially the music circle. He had very limited vision and would hold things very close to his eyes to see them. Roderick could keep a tune well and loved to sing. He could not see the actions of the teacher leading the circle group or those of the other children, so he always sat in front of one of the other teachers. They would whisper what was happening and show him the actions to each song. Roderick would occasionally hum along, but usually he just listened with a big smile on his face, sometimes mouthing the words, but not making a sound. Each teacher in turn sitting with him would try to encourage him to do the actions himself, but without success. When they were not moving his body, he just happily listened. Roderick's mother was surprised to hear this and reported that at home Roderick often sang the songs from school and at times she had seen him do some of the actions.

Why did Roderick not sing or do the actions to songs at school? Why did he always wait for his teachers' touch? Was he just lazy?

The touch of skin against skin often signifies a message such as, 'I'm now in control, follow me,' or 'Go on, do it this way.' The child may then quite literally function as an extension of the adult, perceiving this to be what is expected of him. Could this have been Sally's interpretation of her father's intended touch of encouragement? The pause may have been because Sally was waiting for direction and for her father to take over or control that limb. When it didn't happen, she continued climbing, but could have remained puzzled.

Consider again the significance of vision. Sally's parents were with her. She couldn't see their bodies, their smiles, or the slide. Sally knew the room well and by using her sense of touch under foot or hand combined with her other senses, she could easily have found her way around the room. However, what Sally didn't have was a fully integrated mental picture. Pulling herself up on the slide, Sally was unable to see what would have been visible to a sighted child. In effect, she was operating in a void, concentrating on moving up a wooden slope. Her parents represented pleasure and security.

From this perspective, there was really no reason why Sally should have grabbed hold of her mother's hand. Some blind children might have done so, anticipating perhaps a hug. How was Sally to *know* she was at the top of the slide? She couldn't see the top of the slide or where her mother's hands were in relationship to the slide. In touch with her mother's fingertips, she may have been just as puzzled by this contact as by her father's earlier touches, especially now that both hands were being touched.

After the extra pull to reach her mother, both of Sally's hands were in contact with her mother's fingertips. From Sally's perspective, she had now *reached* her mother. It was quite logical from her non-visual point of view to be poised and ready, anticipating that her mother would make the next move. In other circumstances, this would be normal. When a child reaches out to her mother it is natural for the mother to immediately respond by reaching out to the child. Whether the touch of skin against skin is fingertips or hand is less significant to the child who has never seen. Sally's mother told her, 'Sally, you haven't quite reached the top.' Sally had every reason to be puzzled. The top? To a sighted child, the 'top' in this situation is the visual end to the climb and is *seen* as such from whatever angle it is reached. The normal way that Sally would reach the area understood by her as the 'top' is by climbing with her feet on steps, hands and fingers on a rail, and then moving her legs forward and putting her bottom down on a platform to sit. The situation Sally now found herself in did not match her understanding of reaching the 'top.' Sally is on her tummy on the wooden slope, suspended in space, arms above her head and fingers in contact with her mother. 'You have not quite reached the top' was now a confusing statement. Her father did not understand Sally's hesitation, but his words break into her confusion by giving a very specific instruction: 'Use your arms, Sally, and pull a little more.' This is in keeping with what she had been doing so it is immediately responded to. It is important to remember that *even though a child may be responding appropriately, he may still be confused.* If Sally had the opportunity to repeat this experience a few times, the activity would have been less confusing as she began to understand what she was doing.

Sally, Roderick, and Philip all responded to the message of touch, skin against skin, in an unexpected and unique way. Why each child responded the way he or she did may not be totally understood by everyone.

In this section we are not analysing how the adults could or should have interacted with these children. In fact, each adult acted in a very normal way. To analyse everything said to or done with a visually impaired child would prevent the enjoyment of interaction. It would make relating and communicating structured and formal, and stifle the very joy that is so important to learning in childhood. It is also true that many blind or visually impaired children would not have reacted as these particular children did. What we recognize from these situations is that the touch of skin against skin has implications

for the non-visual child that are significantly different from the implications for a sighted child.

After listening to a similar discussion on the significance of the
touch of skin against skin, one lady who had been quiet for a while
suddenly exclaimed, 'That's it. Now I understand.' She explained,
'Clifford, the little boy I look after, is blind and he has cerebral palsy.
He has finally managed to get onto his hands and knees in the four-
point position. The physiotherapist suggested I put my hand behind
his foot to help him push off, but it doesn't work. Clifford won't
move forward. When I put my hand against his foot, he just wiggles
his toes. Now I know why Clifford doesn't move forward. He's
concentrating on my touch, not on what I'm saying. Instead of giving
the incentive to push off, I am actually encouraging him to stay close,
not move away from me! Until this moment I had never understood
the significance of Clifford being blind. I'm going to put the box of
blocks behind his foot and go to the front to encourage him to come
to me.' We don't know what the outcome was, but we do know she
was thinking clearly. Visual impairment involves so much more than
interesting textures, bright colours, and musical toys.

Author Lois Harral, an experienced worker with Variety Club
Blind Babies Foundation, says, 'Don't let assume loom,' a phrase well
worth remembering. The following example from the book *Can't Your
Child See?* by Scott, Jan, and Freeman tells of a five-year-old blind
child who when asked, 'How many hands do you have?' counted
them and replied, 'Two.' 'How many hands does your mother have?'
He went to his mother and counted her hands. 'Two,' he said. 'How
many hands do I have?' the counsellor asked and the child went and
counted her hands. 'Two,' he said. 'What about your father?' he was
asked. 'How many hands does he have?' The child's father was at
work. 'I guess two,' the child said in surprise.

When referring to a blind child, there are many statements and
assumptions that effectively block thinking through and learning. The
following are three common ones.

I know he knows. This statement suggests it's a foregone conclusion.
There is no need to think any further; you already have the answer.
The five-year-old referred to earlier knew where his hands were,
where to find other people's hands, and how to count. However, this
information did not add up to *knowing* that everybody had two
hands. Certainty that everybody has two of anything comes by visual
confirmation or repeated experience. The statement 'I know he

knows' with reference to a visually impaired or blind child is inaccurate more often than not.

Treat him the same as any other child. After all, he is a child. There is nothing actually wrong with that statement unless it is adhered to when a problem arises. If a problem arises, then the statement is not accurate and will block thinking through and recognizing the difference or uniqueness of the blind or visually impaired child.

Blindness is the least of his problems. This statement is always wrong. It is like suggesting that the child is not the *person* he is. Blindness is an integral part of the child's being. It is not like having cerebral palsy, seizures, burning a finger, or living with missing limbs. It plays an all-important role in the child's learning and thinking process. Every particle of information must be processed non-visually. Psychologist Jean Piaget states, 'Sight is our primary link to the objective world, providing constant information, immediate verification, and allowing elements to be grasped in an already integrated form.' A sighted person's vision is an intrinsic part of his person. It has been estimated that 80 to 90 per cent of all learning is processed through vision.

If a child is visually and hearing impaired, he would be a *deaf-blind* child or, in another terminology, a *multisensory-deprived* child. Whether sighted, blind, deaf, or deaf-blind, each is an integral part of *who* the child is. When a major sense is involved, it affects the child's cognition and cannot be lumped together as 'one of the problems.' If a child is multihandicapped, then the problems caused by these disabilities should be looked at in the light of who the child is – blind, sighted, deaf-blind, etc. – but never as 'just the least of his problems.' Blindness is part of his person, not his problem. To think of blindness as a problem is in effect to disown the very nature of that child. It automatically blocks constructive thinking about the child and thinking through to the solution of any problems the child may have as a result of mental or physical disabilities, or of the problems encountered because he is a blind child in a sight-oriented world.

Many people, including those who are knowledgeable about blindness, have expressed feelings of inadequacy when faced with a child who is blind and multihandicapped. Any child who is multihandicapped is going to present a greater challenge in teaching than a non-handicapped child. However, if the child's *person* is clearly understood (blind, sighted, deaf-blind, etc.), and the perspective is understood, there is no more need to be apprehensive about this child than the sighted multihandicapped child. Greater creativity may be needed and thinking through is essential, but so it should be for all multihandicapped children.

Tuning In and Turn-Taking Techniques

Learning to observe and interact with a visually impaired child is important, but can be difficult at times. Tuning in and turn-taking highlight points that may be helpful to all.

There are people who instinctively tune in and take turns with their child. For most people it is an art that must be understood and practised, and initially may seem difficult. One of the reasons why it is difficult with visually impaired children or blind, multihandicapped children is because so much of our communication is normally through facial expression and gesture. If you have ever felt discouraged about your ability to communicate with your infant or child, *The Secret Life of the Unborn Child* by Thomas Verney, M.D., and John Kelly should encourage you. Your infant or child *wants to communicate with you*. He can and will respond. He was responding to you before he was even born!

Tuning in and turn-taking are worth learning as they help you to develop a deeper understanding of your visually impaired child, and teach you new approaches. One approach is to react to your child instead of always directing him. Many visually impaired children have learned not to act independently because of overdirection. Often they do not initiate because they have not had success in doing so, or the only success they have had has been regarded as negative by an adult.

Consider the plight of a child who is blind and non-verbal because of a physical condition such as cerebral palsy. The child wants to communicate, but can only makes noises. Noises, however, may not generate the immediate reaction of words. The child cannot see if anyone is taking notice. If there has been no acknowledgment of the sound, then the child assumes that no one has heard and so he increases the volume. In all probability, there will now be a reaction, but often only to stop the noise. Stopping the noise may block appropriate communication. To the child the resulting reaction may prove more satisfactory than the feeling of being ignored, and, if so, the child may continue even though he is disciplined. Problems like this can often be avoided when tuning in, turn-taking, and non-verbal communication are learned and practised early.

Learning how to communicate with a child through touch without using words has another advantage. It forces you to relate to the visually impaired child through the non-visual perspective. This approach can be helpful for an older child who is not relating well to words. If a child is behaving in a giddy fashion, this usually indicates that he is reacting more to the interaction and to the sound of the words than to their meaning.

As a training exercise, three teachers were asked to spend a morning communicating with their children through touch without the assistance of words. They found it a challenging and worthwhile experience. They gained an insight into their own actions and their use of words. In the animated discussion that followed, one worker remarked that a child paid attention and really concentrated. Another was surprised to find a child used the limited language she had more effectively, and still another said it was very difficult: 'I couldn't make him understand and we became frustrated. But what really surprised me was that when I stopped talking, he did things that he normally waited for me to prompt him to do.' When you practise and fully understand how to use non-verbal communication you can adapt it to suit many situations, interchanging with verbal communication as required.

The first level of tuning in and turn-taking. You will learn that you can communicate without words and without eye contact. You will also learn how to be *reactive* instead of *directive*. Instead of talking to and touching your infant so that he will respond to you (directive approach), you will learn to wait until your infant initiates a move, and then respond to him (reactive approach). Through waiting and observing you will learn to recognize and react to his slightest movements and sounds. Your child will learn that he has your full attention (vision helps the sighted child know this); that if he initiates a move, he can expect you to respond; and that he can make things happen in a positive way.

While learning the technique, it is best to choose a period when you and the child are relaxed and have plenty of time. Find a quiet place where you won't be disturbed, and hold the infant in a position in which you can both remain comfortable. Be sure he feels secure but not restricted. If you are holding the infant close to your body, he will be reassured by the feel of your breathing. With an older child, choose a cozy corner on the floor or chesterfield and sit with close body contact.

Very gently caress the infant or child's hand or foot. Keep your touch soft, soothing, and consistent. A heavier, intermittent touch suggests a message. A sighted child can see if the touch he felt was accidental or intended to convey a message, perhaps affection, or even correction. For the blind child, every touch is a potential message that can be confusing if not understood. In this case, your touch must not intrude on your child's thoughts. You want your touch to convey the equivalent of eye contact – soft, gentle, and loving. Continue to caress his hand or foot throughout the turn-taking.

Practise being silent. Do not whisper or speak. Wait, be still, be quiet, and watch. Be very patient. In a moment, you will probably feel the child become still. This is the moment when you begin to tune in to each other. Do not break the stillness; continue to wait. Enjoy this moment and wait for the child to make a move. Observe carefully. It might not be his face that shows response. Perhaps it will be a slight squirm or a little noise. When it comes, acknowledge it, but do not talk or whisper. Maintain the stillness. To acknowledge his perhaps very tiny response, you can lightly blow on the top of his head, just once. *Don't take your turn yet.* You are only acknowledging, like a nod in a conversation. You can give a slight extra pressure on the hand that you are caressing – briefly – then return to the soft, consistent caressing.

Continue to wait for the child to take his turn. It may take some time. Remember, he is learning too. The child will probably squirm again or make the sound a fraction louder. *Now it's your turn.* If the child made a small sound, you can imitate it. If not, you can make a small sound yourself. Use touch or your voice (not words). Do not use toys or other sound-makers. Be very still and enjoy this quietness together. Avoid the impulse to hug the child or move. Continue to wait quietly and patiently. He is going to respond in his own very special way. Watch for it. Remember, you have to train yourself to be very observant so as to pick up those first small body movements.

Before you take your turn, always acknowledge his move, however small or insignificant. Your turn will always be a reaction to what your child did in his turn. You can repeat what you did before, or introduce a new special touch or sound. Murmur softly or blow on him lightly, then return to the soft caressing while you wait again. Always keep your turn very short and avoid talking. When your child responds, acknowledge and wait again. This is important. *You must become very aware of the turn-taking sequence. Your child's response is not his turn; it is his acknowledgment of your turn. Be sure to wait until he initiates again. Be patient. Don't become uneasy with the stillness as you wait for him to respond.*

If you have practised the steps described, you will know that you can communicate non-visually and non-verbally. Through tuning in, patient waiting, and observing, you will have learned the joy of communicating in a unique and special way. You will recognize and understand your child's slightest movements as he begins to communicate with you. It is exciting to watch these responses to your caresses and then to see him begin to initiate moves of his own. These moves are the communication base, not only for speech, but also for initiating play. Our hope is that all family members or care-givers will learn and practise this turn-taking technique, then advance to the second and third levels.

The second level of tuning in and turn-taking. In this level, we will teach you the basics of the tap-and-touch method of communication and show you how to use it as an introduction to words. First your child will learn that your touch can give a specific message, then he will be ready to receive added information – specific words for body parts. Be very accurate with your words. You will be building a foundation for language and teaching him about his frame of reference – his body. Do not rush to use words. Be certain that what you are saying through touch is understood. You must learn to make your 'hands talk'. In the same way as your voice has inflexions, so your touch can emphasize specifics. Practise thoroughly before adding words.

As before, make yourself and your child comfortable. This time you will need your arms free. If interacting with a small child, you might lay him on your lap facing you. An older child will need to be close to you, cozy and relaxed.

Choose ahead of time the area of his body you are going to tell your child about. Focus on a small body area and introduce it only during your turn. As in the first level, your turn must always be short. The following sequences are a few of many possibilities:

- hair (A) to neck (B): hair, ears, eyes, nose, mouth, chin, and neck
- elbow (A) to hand (B): elbow, arm, wrist, and hand
- wrist (A) to fingers (B): wrist, palm, thumb, pointer finger, ring finger, and small finger
- knee (A) to toes (B): knee, shin, ankle, heel, and toes

• ankle (A) to toes (B): ankle, heel, sole of foot, and toes

You can choose any small area of the body, front or back, and can include less familiar parts, such as hips, waist, underarms, shoulders. When you change your tapping and stroking, you can include body parts from a previous sequence with the new series of movements you've chosen. Refrain from using words until you are sure your message through touch is fully understood and your movements are anticipated.

Begin by tuning in and use non-verbal communication, as described in the first level. Allow your child to initiate at least twice and respond accordingly. When it is your turn, touch the first and last points (A and B) that your hands will be moving between. Then in one quick movement, slide your hand from point A to B. Now firmly, slowly, and gently, move your hands over the body parts you will introduce. Emphasize with just slightly more pressure the areas that you plan to name. Repeat the tap-and-stroke method as before, remembering to touch points A and B and stroke first. *That's all. You've now taken your turn.*

Now go back to the original gentle caressing of hand or foot as you did when you started. When your child acknowledges, give a slight pressure, indicating that you are still paying attention, and continue to wait for him to take his turn. Even though your child is familiar with the turn-taking process, this time he may be slower. He has just experienced something new in your communication period. When he does initiate his turn, respond accordingly, imitating his sound or acknowledging his movement as you did in the first level. Then repeat the sequence exactly as you did before, and wait again. Remember, do not change. Your message must be clear.

Continue this sequence in turn-taking without change until you know the child is anticipating the moves of your hand between points A and B. Depending on the child and the time you have to practise, this can take a few turns, a few days, or even a week or so. When you can see that your child is anticipating the movements of your hands, you can start to add words. If you have been carefully following the turn-taking procedure, these will be your *first words* in your special communication period, which, until now, has been all non-verbal. As you start adding words, match your voice to your touch. It must accurately simulate your hand movements – slow, definite, but with a warm, gentle quality. At this stage in the turn-taking technique, you and your child should be fully tuned in to each other, so your child will be even more conscious of your words and the quality of your voice.

As before, touch points A and B and stroke. Then *without hand movements*, name the body parts in exactly the same order as you did with hand movements. Name the individual parts slowly, imagining your hands moving as before and speak at the same speed. Let your visually impaired child concentrate only on the words while he remembers the feel of your touch. Now repeat, putting the two together – words and touch. Your turn is over.

As always, wait for your child to acknowledge your turn and to initiate his own turn. Continue to respond accordingly. On each succeeding turn, using the same body area, continue with the same method – touch first, words only, followed by touch and words together. When your child is familiar with one sequence, use the same method to introduce new body parts, but remember to include body parts previously introduced.

Turn-taking remains extremely important. You must always wait for your child's interactions and you must respond to them. The only difference is that because you are being more specific in what your touch is saying, your turn is taking a little longer. Remember, you are both still learning a technique. It is not easy, and you will need to practise. When you see your child anticipating your movements, your enthusiasm may cause you to forget to listen and react to him. This can result in the child's not making the effort to initiate.

When these two levels have been practised and mastered, you will have learned the basic techniques of non-verbal communication. You will have trained yourself to be fully observant, to slow down and wait. You will be familiar with your child's body language. He, in turn, will be tuned in to your movements and be quick to recognize your message. By now, turn-taking should be automatic. You can begin to use this skill in your daily interactions. We suggest that you continue to have your special communication periods. Participating in play, which comes next, should be easy for you.

Third level of tuning in and turn-taking. In this level you will continue using the techniques of tuning in and turn-taking. As you do so, you will learn how to participate effectively in your child's play.

There are three main barriers to interacting with a visually impaired child in play: 1) a rushed approach; 2) forgetting the non-visual perspective; 3) overdirection. Understanding and overcoming these barriers, like the techniques in the other levels, does take practice. Don't become frustrated or give up if some of your initial attempts are disappointing. As before, you are both still learning. Be patient with your child and yourself. Remember, it is just as difficult for you to relate to his visually limited or non-visual world as it is for him to relate to your visual world. Practice makes perfect!

To prevent a rushed approach, make your presence a pleasure to the child and create a calm, relaxed atmosphere. This is very important. Tune into the child. This is still the first essential step. If your child has limited distance vision, try to stay within his visual field. Many times people forget and place themselves out of the child's visual range, which can be frustrating for a visually impaired child. Be close to your child, but first wait quietly and observe carefully.

How do you think the child is feeling? Happy, sad, bored? Is he listening? Watch those hands and feet. Are they telling you something? Sometimes hands are repetitiously manipulating something, but it is the feet that are actually doing the exploring! Perhaps the child's whole body is very still. The child may appear to be only rocking or fidgeting in some way. Perhaps he is fidgeting, or is he listening intently to something? From time to time when concentrating, all of us fidget – doodling, tapping fingers, biting the top of a pen, etc. Immediately stopping undesirable behaviour may not be appropriate now. Wait and continue to observe. Is there something you are not fully aware of? It may be a sound, but not necessarily the predominant sound in the room. It may be something more subtle, perhaps a pen scratching on paper, the click of knitting needles, or a particularly noisy bird outside the window. What exactly is the child doing with the toy, piece of paper, or clothing? Have his fingers found a small bump or a groove? Why is he in that funny position? Has he found an interesting draught or perhaps a smell? Is he using his residual vision? Practise observing and wait. Give the child plenty of time to initiate. Sometimes it may be necessary to take your turn first, perhaps by speaking or giving a prompt to encourage your child to initiate. Be sure you have fully observed so that you can make a good connection to begin the interaction. With a sighted child the connection is often made through eye contact and may be easier to interpret, allowing for quicker interaction. A sighted child will move away or show disapproval if the approach was too rushed for him and made him feel out of control. The difference here is that the sighted child's message may be clearer to us.

The visually impaired child's reactions may easily be misinterpreted. If he is not able to move away, there are other ways of showing disapproval that work equally well. Going to sleep, screaming, throwing things, or demonstrating other types of negative behaviour. An even more successful way is reaching out for a hug, making kissing sounds, singing, saying 'Hi!', or using other diversionary tactics. Remember, you need to tune in to that little person; with practice you will understand where his interest is and make an appropriate prompt or response when he initiates.

Sighted children see the whole at a glance and then may look at the detail. In contrast, visually impaired children must first explore the detail before they can understand the whole. Because he is not able to see the whole, the visually impaired child may not react as expected to a toy or other object and may react very differently than a sighted child. The following example illustrates this difference.

A small group of blind children, from 5 to 16 years old, were given a pair of roller skates to explore. None of these children had ever experienced roller skates. The skates were adjustable in size. They had brightly coloured red wheels and straps. A key for adjusting the size dangled from one of the straps, making a clanking sound when it hit the metal of the skate. What surprised the observer was that the children, with the exception of two who refused even to touch the skates, stopped to examine the same feature. Not the dangling key that made a noise, or the wheels that turned. They passed over the bright red straps with little interest. When his fingers came in contact with the barely discernible raised bump on the skates, each child stopped and ran his finger over the area again, with a look of interest on his face. The bumps were the tops of the bolts that allowed the skates to be adjusted underneath. The visually impaired child finds the detail, unlike a sighted person who may not even notice the bumps. In a sighted person's survey, they would have been just an insignificant part of the whole.

In the section on daily routines, we suggest focusing on specific parts of toys or other objects rather than on the whole. This is one way of recognizing the non-visual perspective, and helping the visually impaired child understand the whole. It might be helpful to refer again to the section on toys. It could give you a greater understanding of your child's play, and help you to recognize what aspects he may be focusing on or perhaps missing altogether.

Throughout this chapter we have stressed the importance of using a reactive approach with visually impaired children. Turn-taking, accompanied by a reactive approach, is also the key to successful participation in play. It is quite possible to react to the child's lead and respond accordingly, and still use your turn to give a new focus.

There is a subtle difference between being directive and giving a new focus. A directive approach is controlling. It allows for little or no deviation. It may block the child's initiative and creativity. *Giving a new focus is interacting cooperatively.* It is like having an animated conversation and throwing out a new idea for the other person to respond to. In contrast, being directive is like someone stating the subject and then dominating the discussion of it. If you have faithfully practised the first and second levels and continue turn-taking you will not be, nor will you ever become, overdirective.

Learning to Interact

Using the example of the children with the skates, we will suggest some possible interaction. We will assume that you have tuned in to the child, which is always the prerequisite to turn-taking, and acknowledged the child's interest in the bumps he found. A very brief comment might be appropriate: 'You found a bump.' This says, 'I am with you and I'm paying attention,' and it adds information, giving the child the appropriate word for what his finger is in contact with. Then wait for the child to take his turn. Many things can happen. The child may repeat the word 'bump' with interest or continue to run his fingers over the bump, perhaps scraping his nail against it. He might pick the skate up and shake it and appear to have forgotten the bump. He has taken his turn.

Take your turn, as determined by the child's action. If he is still interested in the bump, you might try to help him gather new information. Gently touch the child's fingers to indicate that you are going to direct his hand. Then you might say, 'See, the bump is the top of the screw,' as you lightly guide his hand to show him what you are talking about. That is all. You have taken your turn. Don't touch his hands anymore for a moment. Wait for his turn. The child may or may not choose to explore the skate further. It is still important to follow the turn-taking process. It can easily break down at this stage. You want the child to be interested in what you are showing him and may be tempted to force the issue. Don't. Wait and watch. The child may examine the skate and then you can continue in your turn, or the child may change to something totally different. He may even lose all interest and move away. This can be disappointing. From his non-visual point of view, the child has already received a great deal of information and he may need time to assimilate it. When a child loses interest, it can be for any number of reasons. The information may not be connected or understood. He may be in an uncomfortable position or perhaps he feels out of control or overwhelmed. Whatever the reason, always acknowledge it.

Sometimes the turn-taking can continue. For example, you might permit the child to wander off, but continue to play with the skate yourself, making the wheels spin quietly. Talk softly about the key and say that you are putting your foot on the skate, but that it is too small for you. Don't overdo it. Sound calm and be relaxed. Just as a sighted child might observe a situation from a distance, so too a blind child may assess the situation by listening. He may choose to come back after a few moments. If he does, continue playing with the skates, but acknowledge his presence briefly until he initiates and then the turn-taking can begin again. If he does not come back, you can say, 'We can play with the skates another day.' The blind child will have gained some information when he assessed the situation by listening. Your next introduction of the skates will likely be easier.

What steps might have been taken if the child had not been interested in the bump, but was just shaking the skates? The key to your action is always determined by what the child is doing. You would need to wait a longer period to observe. Why was he shaking them? The child may still have been interested in the bump. He may have another toy that has similar bumps and that makes a sound when shaken. If the shaking doesn't stop and he seems to have lost interest – don't be too quick to come to this conclusion – then you will need to be creative. Take your turn by focusing his thoughts back on his actions, perhaps by using the child's words and rhythm. You might gently put your hands against his and softly sing, 'Shake, shake, shake skates, shake skate, shake skate.' That's all. Now stop and wait for his turn. Be patient. The child will probably tune back to you. If you remain relaxed, gentle, and keep tuned in to the child, he will be conscious of your presence. He will feel your companionable, loving attention, not overwhelming and not too directive.

Wait for him to take his turn, then acknowledge it. In your turn, focus on something different, perhaps the key or the wheels. You may sense the child is bored and offer a new idea, such as playing with sounds or words, or you might try a gross-motor activity. Keep it short. You are still turn-taking and reacting.

Through the cooperative approach shown in the three levels of turn-taking, the child will have learned how to make positive things happen. When language has been used appropriately, and is connected and meaningful within the turn-taking sequences, it will be learned as easily and naturally as it is by a sighted child.

Turn-Taking and the Emotionally Fragile, Confused, or Multihandicapped Blind Child

Even though not all multihandicapped blind or visually impaired children are capable of speech, many do reach a functioning level of communication far beyond the expectations of their caregivers. The turn-taking technique takes much time, patience, and skill to develop. For this child, any self-directed body movements may be difficult and some movements are involuntary, making the interpretation of the child's turn more complicated.

Tuning in to the child is essential. The first level of turn-taking may take several months, but given time, the observant adult will begin to recognize subtleties of the child's body language and sounds, and will react to them. Initial progress may be very slow, but as soon as the child catches on to the system and understands how and when to respond and initiate, progress can be exciting. Be careful not to go too fast and become overly directive. The key to success is always taking turns.

Often acting out, self-abusive, and negative behaviours are symptoms of the child's frustration and confusion. Messages given through touch have not been understood. Words and actions have not been connected. Older children usually develop conditioned responses. When turn-taking begins, these responses will have to be ignored, so that the child can learn and understand the new system. The child may require the first level of turn-taking, but, unlike the infant, has more relearning to do. When learning a new language, the older you are, the more difficult it is. Similarly, learning the turn-taking technique will be harder, but by no means impossible. Initially, negative behaviours can be expected to become more frequent as the child tries some of the methods that have worked for him in the past. *This is normal.* The visually impaired child may be feeling very uneasy. His behaviours represent insecurity. Having the adult wait for him calmly, patiently, and lovingly can be an unnerving experience! He will not understand why he is not being directed, why there are no behavioural expectations or demands being made of him. From his limited or non-visual perspective, his whole environment has changed. He has no way of knowing why.

The increase in negative behaviour can make the adult afraid that he is doing something wrong, that what he is doing is not working. He quickly returns to the old and comfortable method and sighs with relief when the child's negative behaviour stops. Turn-taking was not working because the child was still coping with his uneasiness. Tuning in must precede turn-taking. You cannot tune in when the child is acting out, but you can wait it out. As with the infant, it is necessary to be observant. You may be surprised to find that the first initiated response is at the infant level – a slight squirm, a small noise. Wait for him to make his turn a little more definite before taking your turn and proceed as in the first level. *When talking about preparation for a lifetime, does it matter if tuning in and learning the turn-taking takes three days, three weeks, or a year? In our set system the length of time may seem totally unrealistic, but for the multihandicapped and confused child, learning is a lengthy process.*

The greatest problem in dealing with visually impaired children, especially those who are confused or multihandicapped, is lack of time and consistency. There are very few children who do not want to communicate. Turn-taking encourages total communication. It is not intended to reduce negative behaviour or build skills. These become the spin-off benefits as the child and adult build on tiny successes.

Although the adult is initially reacting to the child, it is his responses and initiatives that lead the child on to develop and blossom. Some adults do this instinctively, while others do not, although they may think they are. They tune into the child, are gentle and kind, but they always direct. They are always controlling. For example, the visually impaired child may be given a toy and shown hand over hand how to operate it. He is directed through each step until he can operate the toy exactly as shown. For the child to understand how to operate the toy, direction is necessary. However, if taught through the turn-taking method, over a period of time the adult may be able to help the child explore and find more things to do with the toy that are of interest to the child. This method prevents the child from learning about the toy in a rote fashion, but having no understanding of it. He will be less likely to use the toy for banging and shaking.

Mannerisms

Although we may be unaware of it, each of us has some mannerism or habit. This is frequently more noticeable when we are under stress, temporarily idle, tired, or concentrating.

Mannerisms can be seen in many children when a basic need is not being met. The visually impaired child does not see the many opportunities for spontaneous physical activity that are readily available to his sighted peers – the gate to swing from, the box to jump off, the obstacle-free hall to run along, the hill to roll down, or the puddle to jump into. This lack of visual stimulus causes him to find substitute ways of meeting his needs. Usually, these are body oriented – rocking, bouncing, hand flapping, eye poking, masturbating, vocalizing, head banging, etc. Unless ways are found to prevent or curtail this socially unacceptable behaviour, it can become a habit.

We all know how difficult it is to break a long-standing habit. It is just as difficult for the visually impaired child. He needs our support and encouragement rather than our disapproval. It is difficult for the visually impaired child to understand why certain behaviour, which gives him so much satisfaction, is undesirable to those around him. If the mannerism is to be remedied, there must be understanding and empathy between the visually impaired child and those interacting with him. The first step in helping the child is to decide if there are any periods in the child's day that foster the habit and, if so, what changes can be made.

Do not assume that the child knows what he is doing, even though he may stop momentarily when you ask him. He may be responding only to the tone of your voice. For you to be sure that he understands what he is doing and is not just responding to the tone of your voice, play a game that asks him to do the activity you want to eliminate. For example, sing, 'You rock and you rock and you rock and you *stop*.' Or, 'Can you shake your hands like me? Stop! Let's do it again? Stop! Now you can use your hands to unscrew the lid of this jar and find what Mummy has hidden inside.'

How you help the child will depend on his age or level of maturity. If it is possible, enlist the child's help. Discuss the problem with him. Ask him if he has any suggestions and how you can help him. You could suggest a discreet reminder when he is forgetting; for example, inconspicuously offer him a small stone or elastic band (as well as being a reminder, this provides something to manipulate in his hand) or remind him by whispering a previously agreed-on word. Avoid drawing attention to the mannerism in front of others, which could embarrass the child and damage his self-image.

A firm but gentle physical reminder is sometimes necessary, or make it physically more difficult to continue with the mannerism. For example, a hand on the shoulder can remind a child to stand still, or showing the child how to stand with feet together makes rocking from one foot to the other impossible.

A compromising approach can also be helpful when there is an appropriate place for the child's mannerism. When the child begins to rock he can be told, 'You feel like rocking. Shall we find the rocking-chair so that you can rock?' This method helps to establish that rocking is only acceptable in the rocking-chair. If a child is bouncing, suggest that he use the trampoline or an old mattress you have put on the floor for this purpose. Regular bouncing on a bed would not be appropriate.

A different body position can discourage some mannerisms, especially in very young children. When the child is lying on his tummy with his fists or knuckles in his eyes, change his position. When the infant is lying on his back and moving his head from side to side, roll him over. Alternatively, prop him into a sitting position.

Ignoring the behaviour while involving the child in something more interesting may be helpful. The small child who is spinning around in circles might enjoy putting on roller skates and moving on the carpet from one piece of furniture to another. The young child masturbating might be encouraged to participate in an active game or an activity involving both hands.

Another method is to stop the behaviour and redirect the child to a more appropriate activity. The child who is jumping up and down could be directed to stop jumping and asked to help make lunch. Involve him. He could climb on a chair and reach into the cupboard for the peanut butter or help wash the dishes. The child who is repeating meaningless TV jingles could be asked to stop and be redirected into singing an action song or a made-up song that relates a current activity: 'John is washing dishes, dishes, dishes. John is washing dishes with Mum today.'

Eye poking is especially distressing to parents who are concerned that the eye may be damaged, or become discoloured and sunken. Continual nagging or tapping the hands may only temporarily stop the action while you are with the child. Empathy and understanding will enable you to maintain positive interaction. This will make it easier to enlist the child's help in breaking the habit if it is still necessary when the child is older. We have found no foolproof way of discouraging eye poking. Parents have tried various ways of covering the eyes with glasses, ski or swimming goggles, but usually without success. In our experience, the most effective ways have been methods that keep the child occupied and wanting to please.

In certain eye conditions eye poking may occasionally be necessary to assist the child to focus. It is frequently accompanied by a tilt of the head as the child tries to focus on an object or picture in a book. It is easy to differentiate between this and the repetitious eye poking discussed above.

All of this takes time and patience. Remembering the child cannot see that others are not doing what he is doing, nor can he see the disapproving looks from peers. Do not be discouraged when mannerisms that seem to have been eliminated reappear in times of stress. This happens to everyone and is not unique to the visually impaired child.

Outline for Program Planning

Much of all learning is through vision. It is inevitable, therefore, that all congenitally blind children, whether or not they have additional physical or mental handicaps, will experience some confusion as they try to construct reality without the assistance of vision.

Some children have been confused, but their confusion has not been recognized. Instead the child is thought to be lazy or uncooperative. These children may have inadvertently been taught to be helpless. They do not respond, and act only on a prompt, not understanding what is expected or that they can act independently. Turn-taking and reactive programming, as described in this section, may be helpful to them.

When the confusion is recognized, it can be remedied. The child then continues to build on accurate foundational concepts, and physical and mental development progress to the child's level of potential.

Serious problems can develop when the confusion caused by the mixed messages the child has received is not recognized and corrected. When this happens, the child's basic blocks of understanding may become so fragmented that he has no foundation on which to build. This is the crumbling effect suggested in the analogy of the transparent ball. For these children, the construction of reality is impossible without consistent and appropriate intervention. The world becomes confusing and meaningless, resulting in total conceptual confusion. Such children appear to have a low IQ and function far below the level expected at their age. They may show signs of emotional disturbance, and will likely exhibit many body-oriented deviant behaviours, such as handflailing, rocking, teeth tapping, masturbating. Many of these children become totally introverted and passive, or aggressive with bizarre outbursts, or a combination of both.

For a very confused child, language may be non-existent, echolalic, or prolific but meaningless. To the casual listener, this may be very deceptive, as the child may ream off whole sentences or even paragraphs in story-like fashion. At first hearing, this can appear to be appropriate. However, closer examination will reveal that a two-way conversation with the child at the same level is not possible. These confused children may also have a whole repertoire of songs. As well as their prolific but meaningless language, such children often have some appropriate language, but it is likely to be very basic and relate to bodily needs – for example, 'Mary wants a drink.' The meaningful language will be at a much earlier developmental level than the prolific language the child recites or sings. Some parents report that their non-verbal children said words at an early developmental stage, but are no longer verbal.

In some cases, confused children have skills developed to an acceptable level, but as the skills are not related or connected in the child's understanding to other meaningful experiences, they are used in a robot-like fashion. The child acts as if he has been programmed, showing little or no initiative. These skills can be likened to the disconnected lumps in the analogy of the transparent puzzle ball.

Those who do not have a thorough understanding of the implications of congenital blindness will frequently label such children as mentally retarded or autistic. Mental labelling is damaging if the person doing the labelling is involved with the child's care or future. His preconceived ideas may prevent him from looking more fully into the implications of congenital blindness. The suggestion that the child is very confused and does not understand the most basic concepts, or has concepts that are faulty, seems too simplistic and some other more physiological or academic cause is searched for. Unfortunately, this very search may cause further confusion for the child, who is assessed and reassessed each time with new methods, programs, personnel, and goals.

Concerned parents of such children are under a great deal of stress and have been for many years as they watch their child's behaviour deteriorate and disrupt the family unit. Ongoing assessment and reassessment in a continued search for an appropriate intervention adds to their stress. Fear that custodial care is their only option becomes a constant companion.

The following program outlines relate closely to the sections on communication and preventative and remedial measures.

For the child who is experiencing considerable difficulty in making sense of his world, a special program should be considered. The goals of this program would be to identify and fill in the conceptual gaps in the child's understanding. A minimum of one year will be necessary to provide the stepping-stones to successful integration. Without this type of early remedial action, it is unlikely the child will ever reach his full potential. These are the major factors in setting up a program.

A one-to-one ratio. For a visually impaired child, understanding an adult's touch, words, and expectations is essential if he is to interact effectively. If remedial programming is to be successful, only one person should be interacting with the child for most of the day. This will avoid mixed messages and conflicting expectations. However, a team approach can still be used. Other professionals can assist and support the primary worker, but should not interact with the child. A person knowledgeable about visually impaired children should monitor the program.

The family should make the final choice of a primary worker for their child. It is important that they like the worker and are comfortable with his or her ability to empathize and relate to them and to their child. The most successful worker in this type of programming is not necessarily the most highly trained. The worker needs to be creative, flexible, and willing to think through situations. Common sense, energy, perseverance, and patience will be needed. The worker should be able to work on his or her own, yet be willing to accept direction. Previous experience and a genuine interest in children are necessary, as is the ability to empathize with parents and listen to their concerns. Age is not as important as level of maturity. A cheerful disposition is a must, and a sense of humour a tremendous asset.

A home-like environment. The worker's home may be ideal. It can be quieter and less distracting for the child and more comfortable for the worker than the child's home. In this type of setting, the child can build on the familiar, home-like environment, and gaps in his concept of reality become obvious more quickly. His program should be relaxed and flexible, geared to his specific needs and pace. Activities can be prolonged or changed moment by moment if this proves necessary. His day should be predictable, but without time constraints. For progress to take place, a reactive program is essential. This is not possible when the needs of a group must be considered. A reactive program follows the child's lead, capitalizing on his interests and actions to teach and build information.

Preparation for the worker. The worker is given pertinent reading material on visually impaired children and specific times to observe the child and record observations. Time alone with the family for discussion is necessary, and so is an opportunity to share information with the professional who will be monitoring the program. During the observation period, the worker should remain as insignificant as possible. If introductions become necessary, the worker should be introduced as a friend of the family. Observations should cover a variety of times in the child's day, including any educational or recreational programs he is attending. Here is a guide for collecting information through observation.

- *Visual responses:* Is the child aware of light? Does he choose lit or shaded areas to play in? Does he tilt his head to look? Does he hold objects close to his eyes? See movement across the room?
- *Body awareness:* On request, can the child touch his own body parts and those of others, name body parts, move a body part, kneel, sit, lie on his side, etc.?
- *Body movements:* Does the child roll, shuffle on his bottom, crawl, or walk? Does he favour one side of his body? Is there a dominant hand? How does he use his hands? Are there any obvious difficulties in general posture or movement?
- *Movement in space:* Does the child move purposefully? How does he find lost toys? Can he locate permanent objects? Does he manoeuvre easily in familiar environments, or does he require verbal or tactual prompts? Does he run, jump, climb stairs, etc.? Does he move cautiously or impulsively?
- *Communication:* Is his communication verbal or non-verbal? Does he use words, body language, screams, or specific sounds? Does he use echolalic speech? Does he sing TV songs and jingles repetitively? Can he follow simple directions? How does he make his needs known? Is his talk relevant? Does he listen? How does he get attention? Does he confuse his pronouns?
- *General level of skills:* Is he toilet-trained? Can he dress and undress himself? Does he need pureed food or is he able to chew? Does he eat with his fingers or a spoon?

- *Likes and dislikes:* What are his preferences in music, people, toys, tastes, activities, and sounds? Include anything the child enjoys, even behaviour that may not be socially acceptable.
- *Fears:* Is he afraid of crowds, noise, strangers, animals, equipment that moves, certain body positions?
- *General:* Find out about his sleeping patterns, health, allergies, the names of family members, special friends, pets, and any colloquial terms with which the child is familiar.

Several meetings should be set up between the worker and the child, and these must be carefully planned to focus on the child's favourite activities. They must be kept short so that when the worker leaves, the child will look forward to their next time together. Half an hour is probably long enough. The first few meetings should be at the child's home and subsequent meetings at the worker's home. Activities might include rocking together in the rocking-chair, playing on the swings in the backyard, enjoying a favourite snack, or even a fun bath time (in his own home).

A workshop should be provided by the program monitor for the worker, family members, and all those involved or interested in the child. This workshop should include general and specific information on visual impairment, experiences under blindfolds to clarify points, and discussion regarding the proposed program.

It should be explained that during the first few months the worker and the family will not be relating directly. A logbook will facilitate communication and the program monitor will liaise between the two. Initially this type of program can be stressful for both parents and worker. Although it is educational, it is not as clearly defined as a regular program.

All children behave differently in different situations and with different people. It can take the blind child a long time to understand and trust this new person in his life. While this is happening, his behaviour at home may change. He may even regress. This can be upsetting to the parents. The worker also may develop negative feelings towards the family whom he or she perceives as not being too helpful. He may think the family is inconsistent or not following through with expectations. In the early stages, these are normal reactions. Having a liaison person provides an outlet for both parties and prevents the situation from getting out of proportion.

It should be understood that although the child is happy and settled in the new situation, the worker and the child are still learning about each other, and the necessary trust and rapport is still developing. It has been our experience that it takes fully three months before any significant progress is evident and perhaps even longer if there are difficult adjustments at the beginning.

Building a rapport. At the beginning of the program, the adult and the child get to know each other and learn to enjoy each other's company. Rapport is built through these relaxed and positive interactions. As rapport is the foundation of a successful program, this stage should not be rushed.

Goal setting. The objectives are to give the child an awareness and understanding of his world, and to motivate him to interact meaningfully in his environment. Through the program he will acquire information that will enable him to make some constructive choices and secure some control. During the rapport-building time the worker will have become more aware of the gaps in the child's understanding. Set short-term goals that ensure success.

Detail is important in setting short-term goals. When detail is overlooked, even a simple goal may not be reached. To get a child to use a spoon, the short-term goals would be to interest him in a spoon, to encourage him to hold the spoon while being fed, and eventually to bring the spoon to his mouth.

Tools. Turn-taking, story-telling, and many examples in the activity section, including the appropriate use of music, will provide useful tools in implementing the program and meeting the goals.

Narrowing the environmental boundaries. The purpose is to help the child develop an awareness of his surroundings and build a sound conceptual base. At the beginning it is as important to narrow his environmental boundaries as it is to limit the number of people involved with him.

A limited and organized space provides a more manageable area for learning about the environment. If the child has less space to wander in, purposeful movement is more easily accomplished. For example, the child is more likely to search for a toy he remembers when he knows the toy shelf is only a few steps away than if he must go to a toy-box in another room. The worker will more likely be successful in encouraging the child to come to the table when the child has only a short distance to walk.

The child has to learn about objects in space and where they are in relation to each other. He must also learn to move to a specific object from any place in his environment. He will need to learn the function of objects and how he can use them. When he learns to understand the sounds and tactual clues, moving becomes purposeful. Even though the child may be able to move freely around a large environment, learning about spatial relationships is a complex process and more easily accomplished in a smaller area.

Looking at learning. We gather information through all our senses, visual and auditory input being the most significant. Sighted children tend to be visual or auditory learners. Some sighted children have a lot of difficulty learning through auditory methods. Are there also visually impaired children for whom auditory learning is difficult? If so, their alternatives are limited and learning itself becomes a problem.

Before choosing activities, it is advisable to consider the following types of learning. Incidental learning is gained through casual encounters. Project or situation learning is taking a subject and learning all there is about the subject. Rote learning is counting, learning the alphabet, rhymes, jingles, etc., without necessarily understanding.

When choosing learning activities, it is helpful to decide to which of the three categories the learning belongs. Rote learning is probably the least effective but easiest to teach. If it is used, ensure that the child understands what he is being taught. As we have mentioned previously, meaningless words, songs, jingles, stories, TV commercials, etc., can cause confusion and delay the concept-building process.

Incidental learning can be fun. It is one way of introducing new activities and many common objects that the child may not be aware of before expecting the child to participate fully. Incidental learning should be very low-key and of short duration (one to five minutes). To be effective, it must never be forced. If the child shows interest, fine; if not, try again at another time.

To introduce an object, a useful clue-in phrase is 'Look what I found.' Any phrase can be used as long as it is consistent. Do not force the child's hands to touch the object, for example, a tube of toothpaste. Use the clue-in phrase, then pass the tube of toothpaste with the cap off under the child's nose and comment, 'Smells like mint.' Make it obvious that you are enjoying the smell and perhaps even the taste, but do not ask the child to participate. On another day you might use the clue-in phrase 'Look what I found,' find the tooth-paste, and remark once more on the smell and taste. Depending on the child's reaction, you might take the next step. Say to the child, 'I'm going to give you a little taste on your lip,' put a bit of tooth-paste on his lip and remark, 'Good taste, isn't it?' That would be all. Repeat at a later date, perhaps leaving the toothpaste near the child's hand. This is another example of communicating through touch and words.

It is helpful to have a number of objects ready and easily acces-sible. You could keep each set of objects in separate boxes. Shoe boxes work well and are easily stacked. Cards in the lid with a list of steps for introducing the objects will help you to remember what you had planned to do with each one. A varied selection of objects to use in odd moments between activities is listed below. Use these incidental learning experiences when your child is especially respon-sive. Remember to make connections later by putting each object into a life experience.

- Piece of paper and single-hole punch
- Soap, soap-dish, and bowl for water
- Roll of toilet paper – pull off one sheet at a time
- Box of tissues – pull out one at a time
- Individually wrapped candy or cookie
- Small water jug and cup
- Two jars with lids – small and large
- Band-Aid – unwrap and stick on
- Sunglasses in case
- Padlock and key
- Coins and change purse
- Dollar bill in wallet
- Mitt and glove
- Recorder and harmonica
- Candle and matches
- Brooch in jewellery box
- Toothbrush, hairbrush, nail-brush, and clothes brush
- Music box to wind
- Pencil and pencil sharpener
- Scissors and paper

To introduce a new activity that involves movement, 'One, two, three' has proved to be a useful clue-in phrase. For example, after having walked around the slide, talked in a casual, cheerful way about the slide, and perhaps sat on the bottom of the slide with the child on your lap, take the child to the side of the slide and comment about sitting on the slide. Be sure that the child understands the word 'sit.' Now use the clue-in word and slowly say, 'One, two, three.' (Any words can be used provided they are the same each time.) Then quickly lift the child to sit on the slide and immediately return him to the original place beside the slide. Do not slide him down.

Depending on the child's reaction, you might leave the slide and repeat another time, repeat the action, or go one step further and take the child's hand and slide it down a short way and repeat the clue-in words and, as before, lift the child and slide him a short distance down the slide and immediately return him to his original place.

How a new situation is approached is important. In the above situation, through touch and words, you told the child what you were going to do. A sighted child could have watched the fun of someone coming down the slide. You gave your child a preview of the experience by sitting him on the slide and immediately taking him off. This gave him an opportunity to show his feelings (fear, excitement) and gave you a chance to respond.

Even though the child may appear to be interested and ready for more, it is often better to wait until another time to carry on with this activity. Incidental learning is a good motivator; it builds trust. As there is no pressure, the child is ready and often looking forward to trying the activity again. Always repeat steps and use the same clue-in words before going further. Remember the child does not see the whole and he is learning new details. The trust factor gives the child a feeling of being in control. This gives him confidence to try other new experiences when the person he trusts introduces them.

In situation or project learning, your subject could be a lunch period, exploring the lunch-box or opening sandwiches, operating the cassette player, taking a bath, etc. Refer to the example of Martin in the section on problem solving. His project learning was first the slide and then the other play equipment. He was encouraged to thoroughly explore and experience the slide many different ways.

Rote learning is self-explanatory. All children learn many things by rote and the visually impaired child can usually do this very well. However, he will not understand rote-learned words unless he has some concrete experiences to give meaning to them. Learning songs, rhymes, and jingles by rote can be great fun. In a remedial program for very confused children it is particularly important that they understand the meaning of the words they are taught.

Throughout this book there are numerous examples of intervention techniques that have been used for a variety of children in many different situations. Below there are four more case examples with some intervention suggestions.

Janet

Janet was born prematurely and is totally blind. In some areas she is very immature. Physically she is strong and surprisingly agile. Janet enjoys gross-motor activities. She loves the tire swing in the basement and the climbing frame outside. When so motivated, she will run up and down the steep stairs of her home and move freely all around the house, including going independently down to the basement on her own initiative. Apart from climbing and swinging, Janet does not play constructively. She is easily frustrated and has very limited speech, mostly echolalia. She does have a few meaningful words, but these relate mainly to eating, e.g., 'Juice, cookie, eat,' usually accompanied by banging on the table. There are a few other food words, also 'out,' which means Janet want to go to the climbing frame, and some sounds that her family understand, one of which is a sound indicating she wants her teddy bear. Blind children of Janet's developmental level do not usually take an interest in dolls or teddy bears. Janet does not play with her teddy bear as if it were a baby or friend, but rather trails it around just as some small children trail a security blanket.

Although not advanced, Janet's general living skills are at an acceptable level. She uses a spoon to eat soft desserts, but whenever possible, she will revert to using her fingers, becoming very angry when a spoon is suggested. She locates her cup and drinks from it, replacing it on the table. She undresses with no difficulty, usually not on request and often in very unacceptable places, such as at the shopping plaza, where it is particularly embarrassing, as she becomes furious when prevented. With a little help and a great deal of persuasion, she will dress herself. Janet can be a very lovable little girl, and is especially affectionate with those she knows well. She will either roughly hug or perhaps push away those who are less familiar.

Janet enjoys pinching people or pulling their hair. To her this is a game. She enjoys the resulting squawks from her victims, especially if they do not retaliate. Janet laughs and tries for a repeat performance. This is part of the game. She knows she will be hurriedly pulled away and reprimanded. From Janet's perspective the pleasure of her game outweighs the consequences!

Janet has a much older brother and sister who love to 'baby' her. Their laughs jeopardize their mother's efforts at giving Janet consistent behavioural guidelines. There is no nursery school in the neighbourhood.

Janet is expected to go to a special school for blind children when she is six years old. Before she goes her parents want her to be toilet-trained. Janet is not. Janet's mother has tried everything. Since she was very small Janet has accompanied her family to the toilet. She likes to flush the toilet, and is quite happy to climb up and sit on the toilet – but not if she needs to use it. Janet wets and soils herself. Occasionally her mother hears her grunting behind the curtain in the living-room and gets her to the toilet. Janet's mother is in a dilemma. If she puts Janet into one-piece jumpsuits with a back opening, she wonders if she's defeating her purpose of getting Janet to go to the toilet on her own. Janet has no bladder problems and can hold her urine for long periods. Janet's mother knows Janet should be toilet-trained and cannot understand the problem. She takes her to the bathroom after every meal, but seldom has success. If she sees Janet indicating she needs to go, she very quickly takes her. Janet usually wets before she gets to the toilet, or she wets the seat as she's getting off it. She seldom urinates in the toilet. To make the association, Janet's mother has taken the wet underwear and Janet to the toilet. She has explained, 'Not in your panties, not on the floor, in the toilet.' Nothing has worked.

Janet's brother and sister have started calling Janet a baby and won't let her into their rooms until she stops wetting her pants. They feel Janet is just naughty and should be spanked. Janet's mother is no longer sure. She thinks they may be right. On two occasions Janet wet herself – once when she got off the toilet, and once when she was not far from the bathroom. Janet's mother explained to Janet that she was cross and spanked her. Janet's mother felt uneasy. She didn't think Janet was just being naughty. Janet did not improve after the spanking. If anything, she was worse and seemed nervous.

One day a friend phoned. 'Just saw a book,' she said. 'Train your child in 24 hours. Basically it's role-modelling using a doll.' Janet's mother listened and said she'd try it. She didn't believe it would work. Janet's family had been role-models for over two years!

As her friend had suggested, she put water in the potty and sat

Janet's teddy on the pot. She let Janet feel Teddy on the pot and the water in the pot. 'Teddy's done pee pee in the pot,' she told Janet. Janet's response was totally unexpected. She grabbed the bear, spanked it, ran upstairs, and threw it in the bedroom. So much for that idea, Janet's mother thought.

Later she related the incident to a retired friend who had worked for many years with disturbed children. 'I believe I know Janet's problem,' the friend said. 'Janet thinks doing pee is bad.' Janet's mother objected. 'But Janet laughs when she sits on the toilet and loves to flush it. It's only recently that I spanked her.' 'Nevertheless, I still think that's the problem,' her friend said. 'Try doing nothing for a full week. Janet is not bad or good. Don't praise or scold. Take her underwear to her. Just change her. After a week, tell her she's a good girl every time she pees, even if it's on your good carpet. Don't rush her to the toilet or she may think she's done something bad again. The same when she soils herself. Tell her what a good girl she is. Whatever you do, don't refer to the smell or the mess. Make your family understand.' She laughed, 'Your motto must be "It's good to pee."' In the third week, ask Janet if she can do some pee in the potty or toilet.' Janet's mother was thoughtful. 'It seems strange that after nearly three years Janet wouldn't understand, but you may be right. I know our frustration is showing right now and Janet understands that!'

Four weeks later Janet's mother phoned her friend. 'You were right. It worked. Janet is toilet-trained. She went all on her own twice today. Now, do you have a solution for the hair-pulling and punching? I don't think we'd better tell her she's good.' 'No,' her friend replied confidently, 'but I know we can find a solution for that too.'

Janet's mother's friend would probably have made many of the following suggestions if she were planning a remedial program for Janet. Janet is strong and agile and enjoys gross-motor activities. These should be an important part of her program plan as they provide many opportunities for learning – body awareness and body movements, spatial awareness, and rote learning, such as counting and singing games. Constructive gross-motor activities will provide an outlet for her excessive energy.

Like many blind children, Janet does not enjoy toys. She is also frustrated, perhaps because she is bored and cannot communicate easily. The section on activities can help increase Janet's enjoyment and understanding of her world. Janet has successfully gained attention through inappropriate behaviour. Rather than remonstrate, non-verbal communication can be used. Remove Janet from the situation calmly and without a word. Touch should not convey frustration or irritation. If she feels she is gaining attention, both words and touch can reinforce her negative behaviour. At a different time, story-telling about appropriate and inappropriate behaviour will be an enjoyable way of helping Janet understand.

As well as undermining their mother's efforts to give Janet consistent guidelines, her brother and sister gave her mixed messages by first babying her and later becoming angry at what they considered babyish behaviour.

Wendy

Wendy was blind. She was also hydrocephalic and a shunt had been inserted to drain fluid from her brain. During her first eighteen months, Wendy had been in and out of hospital. The constant changes back and forth from home had caused her to feel very insecure. She was usually tense and irritable with people except her immediate family – parents, brother, and grandmother who lived close by. With her family, Wendy was relaxed and happy except at mealtimes.

Wendy's mother described mealtimes as her 'three-times-a-day nightmare.' Wendy was a small and picky eater, and every meal was a struggle. The only person who had any success was Wendy's mother. Wendy was no better when she was held, so her mother always fed her in the high chair to prevent her from associating an unpleasant experience with being held. Wendy associated the sounds and smells of meal preparation with her mealtimes and immediately tensed. Wendy's mother had tried keeping her in another room until the preparation was completed, but this didn't work. It was as if Wendy felt she'd been tricked. She'd throw a tantrum, arching her back and stiffening her legs, making it difficult to put her into the high chair. Instead Wendy's mother kept Wendy with her. She talked about what she was doing and what Wendy would eat. Although Wendy was still tense and apprehensive, her mother's voice had a calming effect.

One day when Wendy was particularly fretful and her mother was almost in tears, Wendy's grandmother turned on the vacuum in the next room. Wendy immediately stopped fretting, listened, and then smiled. Her mother waited a moment, then continued, fully expecting Wendy to resist. She didn't! The vacuum was turned on again for the evening meal with the same result. That was the first completely happy meal that Wendy had had for many months and it was the first of many more. With the vacuum on, in time her father or grandmother could also feed her.

After a few weeks friends suggested Wendy should be weaned from the vacuum. Her parents disagreed. They believed it was better to build a strong and pleasant association with mealtimes and while doing so develop Wendy's eating skills and introduce her to new foods. Everything was going very well. Wendy was progressing fast. The family were relaxed. Then Wendy's shunt blocked and she was back in hospital.

There was no vacuum. Wendy's mother stayed at the hospital for the first two days and persuaded the nurses to put on the compressor. They agreed reluctantly because it was noisy. Not understanding and because they felt Wendy was being pampered, they suggested a radio or music instead. Wendy's mother was firm. She knew her daughter. 'Please use the compressor,' she said. They did – while she was there.

Wendy was in the hospital for another week. When her mother came to take her home, she found Wendy curled up in the corner of her crib. 'She's asleep,' the nurses said. Wendy was not. When her mother spoke to her, Wendy did not respond, but her mother recognized her body language and knew that she had heard. When her mother tried to pick her up, Wendy clung to the mattress. She struggled and whimpered when her mother tried to put on her coat.

At home the situation did not change. Wendy screamed and fought her family if they tried to pick her up. The vacuum did not help. Wendy's mother couldn't get a spoon near Wendy's mouth and had to put her back on the bottle. She was relaxed only in her crib. Wendy's screaming was affecting everyone. After four days, her mother was desperate. She phoned the agency for the blind. After listening, the counsellor said, 'Wendy must have physical contact. She has to learn to like it again.' 'How?' Wendy's mother asked. 'She won't let us pick her up.' Then she added thoughtfully, 'Do you think my husband's backpack would work? She's now too big for the snugly.' 'If she's not too heavy, try it,' was the advice.

They did, taking it in turns. Wendy's grandmother wanted to help, but was not strong enough to stand with the backpack on. She watched TV sitting in the corner of the chesterfield with Wendy behind her! This continued for a full week. Finally Wendy was willing to sit on their laps, and within ten days she was her normal happy self again.

The family continued where they had left off. With the vacuum on at meals, Wendy progressed well. Gradually Wendy's need for the vacuum decreased. When she was four-and-a-half years old, Wendy went into a regular nursery school and no longer wanted the vacuum except for occasional treats. When she was six she started formal education and continued to do well. Wendy's language was delayed, which slowed her down, and everyone worked especially hard to develop her concepts. By eight years she was reading braille.

Those who are sighted often miss areas that interest the visually impaired child. We need to train ourselves to become aware of these potential aids in programming. Wendy's mother accidentally discovered the benefits of the vacuum in relaxing her daughter. Recognizing her daughter's need for the vacuum, she resisted her friend's suggestion to wean her away from it. She also did her best to provide a similar sound in the hospital. Wendy's mother was wise not to pair an unpleasant experience (feeding) with physical contact. We are often more concerned about doing what is conventional than considering what is right for an individual child.

We are apt to avoid difficult situations, as Wendy's mother did by removing her from the kitchen when the meal was being prepared. In the long run this does not always have the desired effect. It may be better to deal with the situation directly, as Wendy's mother decided to do. This situation also reminds us that the tone of voice is important when interacting with all children, especially the visually impaired child. Although Wendy was very young, her mother could have used simple story-telling and songs to prepare Wendy for hospitalization. A tape of her favourite songs and her parent's voices might have been helpful for Wendy when she was in hospital. It could also have increased her language development.

Pedro

Pedro was a blind five-year-old who had recently arrived in this country. It was reported that he did not speak, was self-abusive, bit himself, and wore a helmet to protect his head when he bashed it against whatever was closest, including people. He hated food; the smell sent him into a panic. Pedro had been force-fed by caring people who feared for his health. He drank from a bottle, grabbing it and sucking at it in a frenzied fashion. He was calmest when curled into a tight fetal position. He was totally introverted to a point where he appeared to be asleep. In fact, he consciously shut the world out and was uneasy when out of his private safety zone. When held in a standing position, Pedro pulled his knees to his chest, refusing to place his feet on the ground and becoming very agitated, flailing the air with his hands and arms and screaming.

Pedro was given a physical check-up and found to be healthy. Professionals were consulted about his disturbed behaviour. Their advice did not take into account the implications of blindness. They suggested that he should be in a small group with other children who functioned at his level. His teacher would concentrate on a feeding program. The physiotherapist, speech therapist, and occupational therapist all agreed they would work with him each week. Everyone was interested in and genuinely concerned about Pedro.

Pedro did not improve. The more people attempted to interact with him, the more disturbed he became. Finally, Pedro's foster mother gave the ultimatum: 'No more. He stays home. We will work with him alone or you take him somewhere else,' she said. The Peles were a retired couple. They knew nothing about programs. However, they knew that Pedro was an unhappy child and becoming more so. It was this that prompted Mrs Pele's ultimatum.

Pedro wanted nothing to do with Mrs Pele or her husband. He would not be held. The Peles decided that dressing Pedro was an unnecessary battle for him and for themselves, so they kept him in sleepers, changing his diaper as necessary. They left the helmet off. Mr Pele had a trolley for moving heavy items. Mrs Pele fitted it with a foam slab and a blanket and wherever she went in the house, Pedro went too.

For the first two days, Mrs Pele didn't attempt anything with Pedro except to offer him his bottle with a highly fortified soup mixture and to change him as necessary. She tried to sit him up, but he grabbed at the trolley and screamed in anger, then remained for over an hour in a tense ball. On the second day Pedro stretched out more, but still refused to be touched. The Peles did not disturb him, although they spoke his name often and made sure he was always close to one or the other of them. They wanted him to become used to the sound of their voices and not feel threatened by them. On the third day Mrs Pele decided that he was calmer and she made some attempts to reach him. She sat on the floor beside him and stroked his head. Pedro grabbed at her hand and bit it, leaving her with tooth marks and a bruise. It took a few moments to recover, then she wound up a music box and placed it near him. Pedro moved away from it and Mrs Pele saw him pulling his knees up tightly and knew he would be beyond her reach, retreating into his own world, if she continued. Later in the day she tried again, but this time while he sucked furiously at his bottle, Mrs Pele gently but firmly took Pedro's foot and massaged it. At first Pedro kicked out and tried to push her hands away with his other foot. She let go, but then repeated the action. Pedro kicked slightly, then gave up and seemed to give his attention to his bottle. Mrs Pele massaged that foot, then let go and tapped the other foot, then massaged it. For about fifteen minutes she alternated from one foot to the other, each time tapping the foot she was changing to. Pedro remained still even after he had finished his bottle; then Mrs Pele left him alone again. An hour later she repeated the process. This time Pedro didn't have the bottle and although he made a disapproving sound, he didn't resist.

The next day the Peles took it in turns to massage his feet every hour, always tapping first to indicate their intention. They were rewarded by seeing him stretch his legs out and relax his arms. They tried once more to sit him up, but he became upset and they left him. They noted he now drank his bottle in a less frenzied fashion. He was definitely becoming calmer.

The following day Mrs Pele repeated the foot massage, but then touched his knee, massaged his foot, walked her fingers up his leg to his knee, and returned to massage his foot. Pedro tensed but didn't resist. She repeated it with the other leg; first tapping the knee, massaging his foot, and walking her fingers up to his knee. She tried touching the top of his leg, but Pedro tensed and seemed agitated, so she stopped. However, by the end of day she and her husband were able to reach his waist by using this technique. Pedro became distressed at any further attempts.

After five days with the Peles, Pedro still wouldn't sit, but he was stretching out and drank calmly from the bottle. During this time he had only had sponge baths and remained on the trolley or in his bed. The Peles were anxious for him to be willing to sit on their knees. Music tapes were not working. They had tried various types, but he always shrank away. Perhaps he associated the music with the efforts people had made in trying to work with him earlier. Then Mr Pele tried something different. He put on a tape of bird sounds and a waterfall. Pedro came to life! He became perfectly still, then sat bolt upright. Mrs Pele brought the tape recorder closer and lifted Pedro on her knee. Gently she touched his hand, then tapped the tape recorder. She then took his hand to the machine. They were all very quiet. Pedro felt the tape recorder and looked interested. He lifted it to his ear. After a few moments Mrs Pele pulled the tape recorder down and Pedro became angry. Mr Pele pushed the button and shut it off. Pedro bashed his head against Mrs Pele's shoulder and roared. Very calmly Mrs Pele tapped Pedro's finger and pushed it against the button; the tape started and Pedro became quiet and then smiled. Again Mrs Pele tapped his finger and pushed it down; the tape stopped. Pedro roared, but didn't move. Mrs Pele touched his finger and didn't push down. Pedro waited and then became angry. Mrs Pele again touched his finger and put slight pressure on it. Pedro understood. He pushed the switch down; the birds sang and Pedro laughed. The Peles were thrilled. Pedro had sat on a knee, smiled, and even laughed. As excited as they were, they did not try to interact with Pedro. Gently, Mr Pele put Pedro back on the trolley with the tape recorder.

Pedro enjoyed sitting on the Peles' laps, providing they did not restrict him by putting their arms around him. He especially enjoyed the rocking-chair. It was many weeks before Pedro would be hugged. With this barrier broken, he became an affectionate and happy child – with them.

Pedro had been very difficult to feed. They had the best success by giving him very small meals several times a day. It was only after he fully trusted them that they were able to have him sit at the table with them. He also learned to eat proficiently with a spoon or fork. From then on, Pedro slowly progressed. He walked around and explored the areas near his trolley. In those early months, Pedro seldom moved far from it. The Peles continued their own tap-and-touch communication with Pedro. Fairly quickly, he began using words, which were always appropriate; simple sentences came much later. When visitors came, he clung to the Peles or his trolley. The Peles encouraged neighbourhood children to come in. This was a very slow process. If Pedro felt out of control he bit, screamed, or pushed them away. The Peles persevered and Pedro began to enjoy the children's visits.

The Peles worried about school. They knew Pedro should go when he turned six. They checked out all the programs and knew he was not ready. A meeting was held. The Peles asked the educational authorities what Pedro would learn at school. They asked for very precise information and in turn explained exactly what they did and how Pedro progressed. After a long discussion, it was agreed that Pedro would stay at home, but that his progress would be regularly monitored by the school. The local agency for the blind also supported the decision.

It worked very well. The Peles had support and Pedro blossomed. At seven-and-a-half years, Pedro went to school. Now the Peles did the monitoring, supporting the school in every way they could.

Although Pedro's foster parents knew nothing about programming, they devised an excellent program for him. They used common sense and creativity to meet Pedro's needs. Instinctively, they recognized that even the most knowledgeable and well-meaning professionals could not help him at this time. They recognized Pedro's unhappiness and were firm in what they believed was best for him.

At five years of age, a healthy child would be off the bottle, walking and running around. Yet for five days the Peles permitted Pedro to remain in his horizontal position. They had one major goal: to establish a rapport. Using the reactive approach, they gave Pedro control. A reactive approach has lasting results, but is very time-consuming and many are not prepared to take the time or willing to give up the directive approach with which they are familiar.

One may wonder how long Pedro would have remained lying down if Mr Pele had not tried the unusual tape. It is a fairly safe assumption that Pedro would not have felt the need to remain in his safety zone much longer.

The Peles did not know how much language Pedro understood. They developed their own non-verbal communication system. Both Peles were able to understand Pedro's body language because they were using the reactive approach, observing and responding to his lead. It is important to provide a safety zone for confused or emotionally fragile children, as the Peles did with the trolley. The Peles were not intimidated by the professionals involved and were able to negotiate an appropriate school program for Pedro.

Grant

Grant is an only child. A visual assessment indicated he could see colour and movement (but no detail) at about two feet. Grant has moderate cerebral palsy and has been in a special program for delayed children since the age of two.

Lack of mobility due to the cerebral palsy and severe visual impairment prevented any degree of spontaneous visual or tactual exploration of his environment. Consequently, Grant's basic concepts are extremely limited. He has had very little opportunity to learn about his family, their activities, and the home routine. His knowledge of school is limited to specific areas of two classrooms.

Grant's parents and teachers are dedicated, caring people. Much time and effort have been given to improving Grant's motor abilities, so by the age of six, Grant is able to walk short distances. As dedicated as Grant's family and teachers are, little real thought has been given to the implications of visual impairment, and so Grant's true potential is not being recognized.

During Grant's four years at school, he has had three different teachers and a variety of teacher's aides and volunteers working with him. People have enjoyed working with him because he is a socially responsive and happy child. For four years Grant has had virtually the same program. Each teacher has used much the same equipment and most of it appears to have little meaning for Grant. Although presented in a slightly different way, from Grant's non-visual perspective it is a variation on the same theme. He cannot initiate or compare visually and the other children are mainly non-verbal. Over the years Grant has learned to respond to tones of voice; he also knows that he is expected to give a particular response or act in a certain way to certain phrases. What skills he has learned are isolated in his understanding. They do not connect to anything that is meaningful to him. For example, Grant can pick things out of a box and drop them in the box, providing the box is always in front of him, which it usually is! He does not see the box, its dimensions, and boundaries. Some one usually takes his hand and says, 'Here's the box, Grant.' Once his hand touches the box, he knows a certain movement is expected from him. If his arm is too far to the right or left when he drops the item from his hand, he expects to hear, 'No, in the box, Grant. Put it in the box.' He does not understand what 'in the box' means, only that he is expected to move his arm a certain distance. Occasionally Grant throws or drops the blocks over the side of the chair. The resulting noise and confusion always delight him.

Grant has a repertoire of words, phrases, and jingles. The only meaning they have for him is the responses he receives from those around him. When bored, Grant says, 'Let's sing "O Canada."' He knows a whole verse and sings it well and in tune. This usually receives an encouraging response. Another equally successful diverting tactic is 'I'm going to give you a hug/kiss.' Grant also knows the most effective way of saying it. His voice can be appealing as he sticks out his arms. He has learned that few people can resist this! These diverting tactics are almost always used during the fine-motor period to speed up the start of his favourite gross-motor period, during which he can practise walking.

Toys have little meaning for Grant, even if they make a noise or have an interesting texture. One toy he likes is the animal noise box. When a string is pulled, an animal noise is produced. Occasionally Grant can be persuaded to use both hands and turn a centre dial to find a new animal noise, but he will not do this on his own, preferring to intermittently pull the string in a repetitious fashion. After he stops pulling it, someone usually speaks to him. He can sit for long intervals with a toy in front of him, providing there is music playing or a great deal of activity going on around him, or if another child is making noises or crying. This especially pleases him. However, if the noise is subdued, he will attract someone's attention by singing. If that fails, banging his head or loud screaming always produces results. If a new toy is put in front of him at this time, he bangs and yells louder or bites his wrist. This almost always results in, 'Better take him out of the chair. Put him on the mat.' Or, if he is very lucky, it could be, 'Put him in the walker for a while.' Sometimes Grant is put in the hall. This too is okay. There is always a breeze blowing – sometimes it is warm air, sometimes cool. Grant usually sings or sleeps. Lunch or snack follows.

After lunch or snack, Grant loves to get off the chair. He also enjoys the praise he receives. He has learned that he cannot get off the chair until he hears, 'Good boy, you're all finished. We're going to ... What do you say now?' Grant responds in his special hopeful voice, 'Get off the chair now?' Sometimes he is asked to repeat it with the preface 'I would like to' and finish off with 'please.' More often than not, 'Get off the chair now?' is sufficient. Grant will often drag out this activity of getting off the chair and revels in the praise and encouragement.

Even though there are children around Grant all day, he cannot see them and seldom has an opportunity to interact with them. At snack time he sits in a regular chair and is close to other children, but seldom seems to be aware of them as people. The noises they make, or their limited conversations, are not different from the sounds he hears throughout the day. For him the food is the only real interest. For a while at potty time he has been close to other children, until quite by accident he reached and found another child's hair. Grant grabbed it and the screaming encouraged him to do it again. He was therefore moved away. He repeated the performance the following day and since then, his chair has been placed where he cannot reach other children. Grant now amuses himself by bumping his chair up and down. This usually brings someone over. If this doesn't succeed, biting himself will.

Apart from the fact that Grant is improving in all gross-motor activities, his overall development changes very little. Grant is conditioned to cues and responds accordingly. He is much like a programmed robot, albeit a happy robot!

A one-to-one program was developed for Grant. In considering the causes of Grant's lack of conceptual development and general progress, it was recognized that he had too many teachers and other adults working with him, and that his program had not reflected the non-visual perspective. It was also too predictable and did not offer any challenges.

His inappropriate communication was accepted as he was a happy and socially responsive child. He was successful in attracting attention by inappropriate behaviour. Putting him in the hall did not help him. It only solved the adults' problem.

It was not possible to provide Grant with an in-home program, which was considered the ideal. The health room in the school was allocated to Grant and the teacher's aide working with him. It offered many of the requirements suggested in the program outline: reduced environment, toilet, couch/bed, hotplate, sink, and refrigerator. The teacher's aide received preparation similar to that described, and many of the teachers in the school attended the workshop. This was a learning experience for all and helped them in their work with other multihandicapped students.

The program was set up using many of the ideas found in this book. Story-telling was used to help develop concepts, new ideas, and appropriate language, as were turn-taking and building on Grant's responses. Many ideas from the activity section were used, including body and action songs. His enjoyment of walking provided motivation for exploring his environment. Games were devised to help him understand spatial awareness. Daily routine activities were used to increase his fine-motor skills, including his favourite – making toast. Because of his cerebral palsy, putting bread in the toaster and pushing down the lever were challenges, but waiting for the toast to pop up and eating it made it worthwhile.

To increase his independence, a small container with cookies or crackers was kept in the cupboard under the sink. Grant was free to have these whenever he chose. As these were favourites of his, he worked hard to open the cupboard door and reach down for the container. This gave him practice in balancing and controlling his movements. Juice was always available, sometimes already poured in a cup or glass. At other times, a juice can was placed by an empty mug (which was embedded in sand to keep it stationary) and Grant poured his own juice. He also enjoyed having juice that came in its special box with a straw.

Grant had never learned to interact with other children. After a few months in his individual program, one or two children were invited into the health room each week for a special activity. These activities were carefully planned. For a few days before his visitors arrived, Grant practised the activity that he would share with his new friends. He learned quickly and in a surprisingly short time he was enjoying the children's company and beginning to interact verbally in an appropriate manner.

As we thought through and wrote this book, we gained a deeper understanding of the needs of blind and visually impaired preschoolers. Perhaps this book has helped you gain a greater understanding of the visually impaired child in your care. We hope you found encouragement and help from the children you met in these pages and from our ideas and suggestions.

Bibliography

Barraga, Nancy. *Visual Handicaps and Learning.* Austin, Texas: Exceptional Resources 1983
- *Braille for Infants: A Preschool and Infant Level Reader Scheme Teachers' Handbook.* London: Royal National Institute for the Blind 1987
Davidson, Ian. *Handbook for Parents of Preschool Blind Children.* Toronto: Ontario Institute for Studies in Education 1976
Gruber, Kathen F., and P.M. Moore. *No Place to Go.* New York: American Foundation for the Blind 1963
Halliday, Carol. *The Visually Impaired Child: Growth, Learning, Development - Infancy to School Age.* Louisville, Ky.: American Printing House for the Blind Inc. 1970
Harrell, Lois, and Nancy Akeson. *Preschool Vision Stimulation: It's More Than a Flashlight.* New York: American Foundation for the Blind 1987
Heiner, Donna. *Learning to Look.* Auburndale, Mass.: International Institute for Visually Impaired 0-7 Inc. 1986
Hyvarinen, Lea. *Vision in Children, Normal and Abnormal.* Meaford, Ont.: The Canadian Deaf-Blind and Rubella Association 1988
Karstein, S., I. Spaulding, and B. Scharf. *Raising the Young Blind Child.* New York: Human Sciences Press Inc. 1980
Kekelis, Linda. *Talk to Me* and *Talk to Me II.* Los Angeles: The Blind Children's Centre 1984
McInnes, J.M., and J.A. Treffy. *Deaf-Blind Infants and Children: A Developmental Guide.* Toronto: University of Toronto Press 1982
Moore, Sheri. *Beginnings: A Practical Guide for Parents and Teachers of Visually Impaired Babies.* Louisville, Ky.: American Printing House for the Blind Inc. 1985

Nielsen, Lilli. *Are You Blind? Promotion of the Development of Children Who are Especially Developmentally Threatened.* Copenhagen: Sikon 1990

Raynor, Sherry, and R. Drouillard. *Get a Wiggle On: A Guide for Helping Visually Impaired Children Grow.* Washington, DC: AAHPER Publications 1975

– *Move It.* Washington, DC: AAHPER Publications 1975

Recchia, Susan L. *Heart to Heart.* Los Angeles: The Blind Children's Centre 1985

– *Welcome to the World.* Los Angeles: The Blind Children's Centre 1985

Robinet, Judy M. *A Life Worth Living: A Book about Parenting Infants and Preschoolers with Visual Impairment and Multidisability.* Windsor, Ont.: Robinet Publications 1992

Santin, Sylvia, and J.N. Simmons. 'Problems in the Construction of Reality in Congenitally Blind Children.' In *Visual Impairment and Blindness*, 72 (December 1978): 425–9

Scott, Eileen P., J.E. Jan, and R.D. Freeman. *Can't Your Child See?* Austin, Tex.: Pro-Ed Press 1985

Smith, Audrey, and Karen Shane Cote. *Look at Me.* Philadelphia, Pa.: Pennsylvania College of Optometry Press 1982

Terrell, Kay Alicyn. *Parenting Preschoolers: Suggestions for Raising Young Blind and Visually Impaired Children.* New York: American Foundation for the Blind 1984

– *Reach Out and Teach.* New York: American Foundation for the Blind 1985

– *The Visually Impaired Child in Hospital*, 2nd ed. Toronto: Ontario Foundation for Visually Impaired Children Inc. 1992

Webster, Richard. *The Road to Freedom: A Parent's Guide to Prepare the Blind Child to Travel Independently.* Jacksonville, Ill.: Katan Publications 1977

Index

behaviour, 103, 211–12; disturbing, 79, 80, 101–2, 237–42, 249–62; manipulative, 25–6; response to pain, 79
body awareness, 73–7, 83, 93–4, 115–16, 120, 121, 144–51; games for promoting, 156, 159, 188–9; stories for promoting, 199–202
books, 135–7
braille, 215

careers, 20–2
challenges, 53–7
communication, 57–73, 84–9, 94–5, 97–100, 192–3, 211, 226–37, 244, 254–8; overwhelming, 60, 86; story-telling, 194–204
comparisons, 73–81, 126, 141
concept development, 57–8, 89–90, 130–3, 138–42, 189–92, 218–26, 258–62; relating to the body, 93–4; confused, 240–2, 258–62; games and crafts for promoting, 152–87; music for promoting, 144–51; relating to representations, 89, 129, 136; story-telling for promoting, 194–204; relating to visual language, 69–71, 103–5
constipation, 30

daily living skills, 120, 241; bathing, 119, 141; dressing, 32–4, 42, 119; eating, 30–2, 42, 118, 202, 214, 221; household tasks, 138–42; sleeping, 35–9; toileting, 34–5, 249–52
definitions (blind, visually impaired, partially sighted), 4

environment, 43–8
exploration, 43, 189–91

family, 8, 28–9
feelings, 8–15, 24–5, 27–8, 105–6, 241; understanding of, 52, 53
fine motor, 116–17, 124–6, 132–3, 163, 165–86

gross motor, 83, 121–4, 130–1, 133–5, 188–93, 220–1, 224
growth, 76, 121, 139
guide dogs, 141

hobbies, 127
hospitalization, 142–3, 252–4; preparing for pain, 79

imitation, 42–3
independence, 6–7, 81–2, 100

language development, 57–73, 97, 127–8, 219; echolalia, 86–7, 97, 241; non-verbal, 64, 67, 241, 254–8; words and rhymes for promoting, 65–6, 147
laziness, 40–1, 221–2, 240
learning: process of, 43–8, 216–18, 233, 246–9; through challenge, 54; through enjoyment, 51

mannerisms, 51, 71–2, 237–40
mistakes, 22–3, 52–3
mixed messages, 50–3
mobility, 16–18, 55–7, 122–4, 207, 224
motivation, 57, 69, 102; through challenge, 55–7; through information, 50; through music, 52; through vision, 44, 110
multihandicapped, 19, 64, 91, 145, 225–6, 236–7, 258–62
music, 97–100, 144–51; as background, 98; games, 152–6, 159; inappropriate use of, 50–1, 65

object permanence, 49

observation, 67–8, 111, 114–16, 232–3, 243–4

pets, 141
play: imaginatively, 126, 141; outdoor, 214–15; with sand, 127; with water, 126–7, 161
problem solving, 48–53

responses: honest feedback, 22, 23, 81, 88; to questions re visual impairment, 24–5, 105–6

sensory, 43–8, 96–7, 120–1, 127–30, 191, 193, 200–1, 218–23, 252–4
sexuality, abuse, 78–9; education, 73–81, 207
socialization, 64, 69, 97, 98, 105–6, 142; crafts to promote, 173–6; games to promote, 152–65
spatial awareness, 94–6, 100, 189–92
stubbornness, 40–1, 221–2, 240

tactile defensive, 102–3, 125
toilet training, 34–5, 42, 249–52
toys, 39–40

vision: child's understanding of, 24, 48; colour, 104; conditions affecting, 18–19; seizures, 114; stimulation, 110–14; understanding eye condition, 41, 90–2; use of blindfolds, 27; use of vision, 92–3